Nursing Research Using Historical Methods

Mary de Chesnay, PhD, RN, PMHCNS-BC, FAAN, is professor at Kennesaw State University, School of Nursing, Kennesaw, Georgia. She has received 13 research grants and has authored two books: *Sex Trafficking: A Clinical Guide for Nurses* (Springer Publishing) and the AJN Book of the Year Award winner, *Caring for the Vulnerable: Perspectives in Nursing Theory, Practice and Research*, now in its third edition (with a fourth edition to be published in 2015). Dr. de Chesnay has published over 21 journal articles in *Qualitative Health Research, Journal of Nursing Management, International Journal of Medicine & Law,* and others. A former dean and endowed chair, she reviews for a variety of professional journals. Dr. de Chesnay is a noted expert on qualitative research and a founding member and first vice president of the Southern Nursing Research Society.

Nursing Research Using Historical Methods

Qualitative Designs and Methods in Nursing

Mary de Chesnay, PhD, RN, PMHCNS-BC, FAAN

Editor

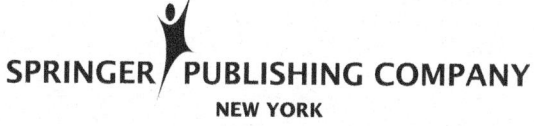

SPRINGER PUBLISHING COMPANY

NEW YORK

Copyright © 2015 Springer Publishing Company, LLC

All rights reserved.

No part of this publication may be reproduced, stored in a retrieval system, or transmitted in any form or by any means, electronic, mechanical, photocopying, recording, or otherwise, without the prior permission of Springer Publishing Company, LLC, or authorization through payment of the appropriate fees to the Copyright Clearance Center, Inc., 222 Rosewood Drive, Danvers, MA 01923, 978-750-8400, fax 978-646-8600, info@copyright.com or on the Web at www.copyright.com.

Springer Publishing Company, LLC
11 West 42nd Street
New York, NY 10036
www.springerpub.com

Acquisitions Editor: Joseph Morita
Production Editor: Kris Parrish
Composition: Exeter Premedia Services Private Ltd.

ISBN: 978-0-8261-2617-7
e-book ISBN: 978-0-8261-2618-4

Set ISBN: 978-0-8261-7134-4
Set e-book ISBN: 978-0-8261-3015-0

14 15 16 17 / 5 4 3 2 1

The author and the publisher of this Work have made every effort to use sources believed to be reliable to provide information that is accurate and compatible with the standards generally accepted at the time of publication. Because medical science is continually advancing, our knowledge base continues to expand. Therefore, as new information becomes available, changes in procedures become necessary. We recommend that the reader always consult current research and specific institutional policies before performing any clinical procedure. The author and publisher shall not be liable for any special, consequential, or exemplary damages resulting, in whole or in part, from the readers' use of, or reliance on, the information contained in this book. The publisher has no responsibility for the persistence or accuracy of URLs for external or third-party Internet websites referred to in this publication and does not guarantee that any content on such websites is, or will remain, accurate or appropriate.

Library of Congress Cataloging-in-Publication Data
Nursing research using historical methods : qualitative designs and methods in nursing / [edited by] Mary de Chesnay.
   p. ; cm.
   Includes bibliographical references.
   ISBN 978-0-8261-2617-7—ISBN 978-0-8261-2618-4 (e-book)
   I. de Chesnay, Mary, editor.
   [DNLM: 1. Nursing Research—methods. 2. Biography as Topic. 3. Historiography.
   4. Interviews as Topic. 5. Qualitative Research. WY 20.5]
   RT81.5
   610.73072—dc23
                                                                                            2014032739

Special discounts on bulk quantities of our books are available to corporations, professional associations, pharmaceutical companies, health care organizations, and other qualifying groups. If you are interested in a custom book, including chapters from more than one of our titles, we can provide that service as well.

For details, please contact:
Special Sales Department, Springer Publishing Company, LLC
11 West 42nd Street, 15th Floor, New York, NY 10036-8002
Phone: 877-687-7476 or 212-431-4370; Fax: 212-941-7842
E-mail: sales@springerpub.com

Printed in the United States of America by Gasch Printing.

QUALITATIVE DESIGNS AND METHODS IN NURSING

Mary de Chesnay, PhD, RN, PMHCNS-BC, FAAN, Series Editor

Nursing Research Using Ethnography: Qualitative Designs and Methods in Nursing

Nursing Research Using Grounded Theory: Qualitative Designs and Methods in Nursing

Nursing Research Using Life History: Qualitative Designs and Methods in Nursing

Nursing Research Using Phenomenology: Qualitative Designs and Methods in Nursing

Nursing Research Using Historical Methods: Qualitative Designs and Methods in Nursing

Nursing Research Using Participatory Action Research: Qualitative Designs and Methods in Nursing

Nursing Research Using Data Analysis: Qualitative Designs and Methods in Nursing

For my nephew, Matt, who will probably be reincarnated as a cat. For my honorary nephew, Chris, whose current incarnation is as a free spirit.
—MdC

Contents

Contributors ix
Foreword Lynda P. Nauright, EdD, RN *xiii*
Series Foreword *xv*
Preface *xxi*
Acknowledgments *xxiii*

1 Learning the Historical Method: Step by Step 1
   Sandra B. Lewenson and Annemarie McAllister

2 Essay on Sources 23
   Patricia D'Antonio
   Commentary: Interview With Dr. Barbra Mann Wall
   Mary de Chesnay

3 Inside Track of Doing Historical Research: My Dissertation Story 41
   Annemarie McAllister and Sandra B. Lewenson

4 History in the Making: Organizing a Nursing History Dissertation 59
   Jeannine Uribe

5 Conducting Oral History Research in Community Mental Health Nursing 85
   Geertje Boschma

6 Celluloid Angels: The Power of Stories 105
   David Stanley

7 The Navajo Experience of Elizabeth Forster, Public Health Nurse 121
   Mary Ann Ruffing-Rahal

8   Sojourner: Life Stories of a Global Health Nurse   *137*
    Barbara A. Anderson

9   Aviation Pioneers: World War II Air Evacuation Nurses   *175*
    Susan Y. Stevens
    Commentary: History Through the Lens of a Nurse
    Susan Y. Stevens

Appendix A   List of Journals That Publish Qualitative Research   *191*
               Mary de Chesnay

Appendix B   Essential Elements for a Qualitative Proposal   *195*
               Tommie Nelms

Appendix C   Writing Qualitative Research Proposals   *197*
               Joan L. Bottorff

Appendix D   Outline for a Research Proposal   *205*
               Mary de Chesnay

Index   209

Contributors

Barbara A. Anderson, Dr PH, RN, CNM, FACNM, FAAN, is professor of nursing and director of the post-master's doctor of nursing practice (DNP) program at Frontier Nursing University. She serves on the board of directors of the American College of Nurse Midwives. She has worked in over 100 countries in public health, nurse-midwifery, program design, and evaluation and education of health professionals.

Geertje Boschma, PhD, RN, is associate professor of nursing at the University of British Columbia, Vancouver, Canada. She has conducted research on the history of nursing and mental health care in the Netherlands, the United States, and Canada. Recent studies by Dr. Boschma have examined the development of community mental health service and general hospital psychiatry in the latter half of the 20th century. She has taught courses in undergraduate and graduate nursing programs on mental health, foundational nursing theory, nursing history, and philosophy.

Joan L. Bottorff, PhD, RN, FCAHS, FAAN, is professor of nursing at the University of British Columbia, Okanagan campus, faculty of Health and Social Development. She is the director of the Institute for Healthy Living and Chronic Disease Prevention at the University of British Columbia.

Patricia D'Antonio, PhD, EN, FAAN, is professor of nursing at the University of Pennsylvania, where she is also the chair of the Department of Family and Community Health and a senior fellow at the Leonard Davis Institute of Health Economics. Dr. D'Antonio is also the author of *American Nursing: A History of Knowledge, Authority and the Meaning of Work* (2010) and editor of the *Nursing History Review*, the official journal of the American Association for the History of Nursing.

Mary de Chesnay, PhD, RN, PMHCNS-BC, FAAN, is professor of nursing at Kennesaw State University and secretary of the Council on Nursing and Anthropology (CONAA) of the Society for Applied Anthropology (SFAA). She has conducted ethnographic fieldwork and participatory action research in Latin America and the Caribbean. She has taught qualitative research at all levels in the United States and abroad in the roles of faculty, head of a department of research, dean, and endowed chair.

Sandra B. Lewenson, EdD, RN, FAAN, is professor of nursing at the Lienhard School of Nursing, College of Health Professions, Pace University, Pleasantville, New York. She has conducted historical research on nursing's role in public health, nursing education, and political activism throughout the early and mid-20th century. She also has taught courses in nursing history and historical methodology, as well as methods used to integrate historical research in all levels of the nursing curriculum.

Annemarie McAllister, EdD, RN, is adjunct assistant professor of nursing at the Lienhard School of Nursing, College of Health Professions, Pace University, Pleasantville, New York. She has taught leadership courses at the graduate level as well as nursing history at the undergraduate level. Her research interests include the development of nursing education in the mid-20th century in the United States and the role of nurse leaders in the development of the associate degree model for the education of nurses. Dr. McAllister also manages a Columbia University cardiology practice in White Plains, New York.

Tommie Nelms, PhD, RN, is professor of nursing at Kennesaw State University. She is director of the WellStar School of Nursing and coordinator of the Doctor of Nursing Science program. She has a long history of conducting and directing phenomenological research and has been a student of Heideggerian philosophy and research for many years. Her research is mainly focused on practices of mothering, caring, and family.

Mary Ann Ruffing-Rahal, PhD, RN, is an associate professor at Ohio State University in Columbus, Ohio.

David Stanley, NursD, MSc HS, BA Ng, DipHE (Nursing), RN, RM, Grad. Cert. HPE, Gerontic Cert., began his nursing career in the days when nurses wore huge belt buckles and funny hats. He is currently an associate professor at the University of Western Australia and has undertaken a number of qualitative studies using grounded theory and phenomenology. He has also undertaken a number of mixed methods studies with a more pragmatic approach to data collection and analysis. David has taught research methods to undergraduate and postgraduate nursing and allied health students at a number of universities in Australia and Asia and supervised a number of higher degree research students to successful completion.

Susan Y. Stevens, PhD, APRN, PMHCNS-BC, is programs chair at Perimeter Adult Learning and Services. She has been a professor, clinician, and researcher. Her research has spanned qualitative and quantitative methods. She has focused particularly on images of nursing in the media and has taught courses in nursing and media for undergraduate and graduate nursing students.

Jeannine Uribe, PhD, RN, is an assistant clinical professor of nursing at Drexel University College of Nursing and Health Professions. She has taught research courses to graduates and undergraduates online and in the classroom. She is currently a board member of the Museum of Nursing History, Inc., in Philadelphia, where she continues to assist nurses to preserve and view their heritage.

Foreword

Nursing researchers, practitioners of nursing, and nursing theorists have long debated whether nursing is a verb, indicating action, or a noun, signifying knowledge. Arguments can and have been made articulately that nursing is an art, a science, and even a calling. Is nursing what nurses do or what nurses know? For the graduate student anticipating hours of coursework, stacks of scholarly papers, and a thesis or project looming on the horizon, these questions are of about as much interest as faculty members' obsession with whether anal-retentive needs a hyphen. The editor of this book recognizes that.

My academic career started with a brief stint as an instructor in an associate degree program attended mostly by licensed practical nurses, followed by a valiant attempt to coordinate a baccalaureate degree completion program for experienced registered nurses. In both cases, students were mostly older and more experienced in nursing than I was. And in both cases they questioned, sometimes vehemently, why they should study a profession they already knew how to do just for the sake of a piece of paper.

My solution to the problem was to try to convince them that knowing how to do something was not the same as *understanding* something. For their first assignment, I asked them to define nursing practice, nursing theory, and nursing research, and to schematically illustrate how these were related to each other. Obviously, I was not expecting one particular outcome and all attempts were equally rewarded, although they varied widely in creativity and depth. The purpose of the assignment was to convince them that just because they could do nursing tasks, they were not as knowledgable as they needed to be about the profession. I was trying to implant the idea that we must *know* more so that we can *do* better.

Historical research is critical to understanding nursing and what nurses do. Optimal nursing practice requires integration of scientific knowledge with knowledge gained through reflection and relationship. Historical research helps us to reclaim and value the comprehensive views of early nurses who intuitively (perhaps unscientifically, perhaps not) practiced in egocentric, homocentric, and ecocentric environmental paradigms, emerging into what has been called the transpersonal caring–healing model.

This series of texts in qualitative design gives guidance and encouragement to fledgling researchers to acknowledge, value, and learn from the voices of nurses from the past. I once interviewed a 96-year-old Black public health nurse who practiced in the 1940s. When I asked her about her career in nursing, she said, "Honey, I didn't have a career; I just had a job. All they wanted was my hands, they could have had my head and my heart for free." We need to record, distribute, and value what is in the heads and hearts of nurses so that we can *do* better. This book helps us learn, not only *how*, but *why*.

Lynda P. Nauright, EdD, RN
Professor Emeritus, Emory University
Atlanta, Georgia

SERIES FOREWORD

In this section, which is published in all volumes of the series, we discuss some key aspects of any qualitative design. This is basic information that might be helpful to novice researchers or those new to the designs and methods described in each chapter. The material is not meant to be rigid and prescribed because qualitative research by its nature is fluid and flexible; the reader should use any ideas that are relevant and discard any ideas that are not relevant to the specific project in mind.

Before beginning a project, it is helpful to commit to publishing it. Of course, it will be publishable because you will use every resource at hand to make sure it is of high quality and contributes to knowledge. Theses and dissertations are meaningless exercises if only the student and committee know what was learned. It is rather heart-breaking to think of all the effort that senior faculty have exerted to complete a degree and yet not to have anyone else benefit by the work. Therefore, some additional resources are included here. Appendix A for each book is a list of journals that publish qualitative research. References to the current nursing qualitative research textbooks are included so that readers may find additional material from sources cited in those chapters.

FOCUS

In qualitative research the focus is emic—what we commonly think of as "from the participant's point of view." The researcher's point of view, called "the etic view," is secondary and does not take precedence over what the participant wants to convey, because in qualitative research, the focus is on the person and his or her story. In contrast, quantitative researchers take pains to learn as much as they can about a topic and focus the research data collection on what they want to know. Cases or subjects that do not provide information about the researcher's agenda are considered outliers and are discarded or treated as aberrant data. Qualitative researchers embrace outliers and actively seek diverse points of view from participants to enrich the data. They sample for diversity within groups and welcome different perceptions even if they seek fairly homogenous samples. For example, in Leenerts and Magilvy's (2000) grounded theory study to examine self-care practices among women, they narrowed the study to low-income, White, HIV-positive women but included both lesbian and heterosexual women.

PROPOSALS

There are many excellent sources in the literature on how to write a research proposal. A couple are cited here (Annersten, 2006; Mareno, 2012; Martin, 2010; Schmelzer, 2006), and examples are found in Appendices B, C, and D. Proposals for any type of research should include basic elements about the purpose, significance, theoretical support, and methods. What is often lacking is a thorough discussion about the rationale. The rationale is needed for the overall design as well as each step in the process. Why qualitative research? Why ethnography and not phenomenology? Why go to a certain setting? Why select the participants through word of mouth? Why use one particular type of software over another to analyze data?

Other common mistakes are not doing justice to significance and failure to provide sufficient theoretical support for the approach. In qualitative research, which tends to be theory generating instead of theory testing, the author still needs to explain why the study is conducted from a particular frame of reference. For example, in some ethnographic work, there are hypotheses that are tested based on the work of prior ethnographers who studied that culture, but there is still a need to generate new theory about current phenomena within that culture from the point of view of the specific informants for the subsequent study.

Significance is underappreciated as an important component of research. Without justifying the importance of the study or the potential impact of the study, there is no case for why the study should be conducted. If a study cannot be justified, why should sponsors fund it? Why should participants agree to participate? Why should the principal investigator bother to conduct it?

COMMONALITIES IN METHODS

Interviewing Basics

One of the best resources for learning how to interview for qualitative research is by Patton (2002), and readers are referred to his book for a detailed guide to interviewing. He describes the process, issues, and challenges in a way that readers can focus their interview in a wide variety of directions that are flexible, yet rigorous. For example, in ethnography, a mix of interview methods is appropriate, ranging from unstructured interviews or informal conversation to highly structured interviews. Unless nurses are conducting mixed-design studies, most of their interviews will be semistructured. Semistructured interviews include a few general questions, but the interviewer is free to allow the interviewee to digress along any lines he or she wishes. It is up to the interviewer to bring the interview back to the focus of the research. This requires skill and sensitivity.

Some general guidelines apply to semistructured interviews:

- Establish rapport.
- Ask open-ended questions. For example, the second question is much more likely to generate a meaningful response than the first in a grounded theory study of coping with cervical cancer.

    Interviewer: Were you afraid when you first heard your diagnosis of cervical cancer?

    Participant: Yes.

  Contrast the above with the following:

    Interviewer: What was your first thought when you heard your diagnosis of cervical cancer?

    Participant: I thought of my young children and how they were going to lose their mother and that they would grow up not knowing how much I loved them.

- Continuously "read" the person's reactions and adapt the approach based on response to questions. For example, in the interview about coping with the diagnosis, the participant began tearing so the interviewer appropriately gave her some time to collect herself. Maintaining silence is one of the most difficult things to learn for researchers who have been classically trained in quantitative methods. In structured interviewing, we are trained to continue despite distractions and to eliminate bias, which may involve eliminating emotion and emotional reactions to what we hear in the interview. Yet the quality of outcomes in qualitative designs may depend on the researcher–participant relationship. It is critical to be authentic and to allow the participant to be authentic.

Ethical Issues

The principles of the Belmont Commission apply to all types of research: respect, justice, beneficence. Perhaps these are even more important when interviewing people about their culture or life experiences. These are highly personal and may be painful for the person to relate, though I have found that there is a cathartic effect to participating in naturalistic research with an empathic interviewer (de Chesnay, 1991, 1993).

Rigor

Readers are referred to the classic paper on rigor in qualitative research (Sandelowski, 1986). Rather than speak of validity and reliability we use other terms, such as accuracy (Do the data represent truth as the participant sees it?) and replicability (Can the reader follow the decision trail to see why the researcher concluded as he or she did?).

DATA ANALYSIS

Analyzing data requires many decisions about how to collect data and whether to use high-tech measures such as qualitative software or old-school measures such as colored index cards. The contributors to this series provide examples of both.

Mixed designs require a balance between the assumptions of quantitative research while conducting that part and qualitative research during that phase. It can be difficult for novice researchers to keep things straight. Researchers are encouraged to learn each paradigm well and to be clear about why they use certain methods for their purposes. Each type of design can stand alone, and one should never think that qualitative research is *less than* quantitative; it is just different.

Mary de Chesnay

REFERENCES

Annersten, M. (2006). How to write a research proposal. *European Diabetes Nursing, 3*(2), 102–105.

de Chesnay, M. (1991, March 13–17). *Catharsis: Outcome of naturalistic research.* Presented to Society for Applied Anthropology, Charleston, SC.

de Chesnay, M. (1993). Workshop with Dr. Patricia Marshall of Symposium on Research Ethics in Fieldwork. Sponsored by Society for Applied Anthropology, Committee on Ethics. Memphis, March 25–29, 1992; San Antonio, Texas, March 11–14, 1993.

Leenerts, M. H., & Magilvy, K. (2000). Investing in self-care: A midrange theory of self-care grounded in the lived experience of low-income HIV-positive white women. *Advances in Nursing Science, 22*(3), 58–75.

Mareno, N. (2012). Sample qualitative research proposal: Childhood obesity in Latino families. In M. de Chesnay & B. Anderson (Eds.), *Caring for the vulnerable* (pp. 203–218). Sudbury, MA: Jones and Bartlett.

Martin, C. H. (2010). A 15-step model for writing a research proposal. *British Journal of Midwifery, 18*(12), 791–798.

Patton, M. Q. (2002). *Qualitative research and evaluation methods* (3rd ed.). Thousand Oaks, CA: Sage.

Sandelowski, M. (1986). The problem of rigor in qualitative research. *Advances in Nursing Science, 4*(3), 27–37.

Schmelzer, M. (2006). How to start a research proposal. *Gastroenterology Nursing, 29*(2), 186–188.

Preface

Qualitative research has evolved from a slightly disreputable beginning to wide acceptance in nursing research. Approaches that focus on the stories and perceptions of the people, instead of what scientists think the world is about, have been a tradition in anthropology for a long time and have created a body of knowledge that cannot be replicated in the lab. The richness of human experience is what qualitative research is all about. Respect for this tradition was long in coming among the scientific community. Nurses seem to have been in the forefront, and though many of my generation (children of the 1950s and 1960s) were classically trained in quantitative techniques, we found something lacking. Perhaps because I am a psychiatric nurse, I have been trained to listen to people tell me their stories, whether the stories are problems that nearly destroy the spirit, or uplifting accounts of how they live within their cultures, or how they cope with terrible traumas and chronic diseases. It seems logical to me that a critical part of developing new knowledge that nurses can use to help patients is to find out first what the patients themselves have to say.

Series volumes address ethnography, grounded theory, life history, phenomenology, historical research, participatory action research, and data analysis. Efforts have been made to recruit contributors from several countries in order to demonstrate global applicability of qualitative research. There are many fine textbooks on nursing research that provide an overview of all the methods, but our aim here is to provide specific information to guide graduate students and experienced nurses who are novices in the designs represented in this series in conducting studies from the point of view of our constituents—patients and their families.

The chapters in this volume on historical research reflect the array of methods including autobiography, biography, oral history, and document review. The authors are experts in collecting historical data and their first-person accounts convey the richness of the designs. I was involved in only two oral history studies, one as an exercise in graduate school in which I interviewed my elderly aunt, a former tuberculosis nurse, who had stories not only of the early days of working in a sanatorium, but also about being a nurse in the early 1900s and helping a physician perform an appendectomy on a farmhouse kitchen table with only moonshine for anesthesia. The second project was to encourage my father, a veteran of the cavalry in World War II, to participate in the oral history project of the Veterans History Project of the American Folklife Center.

The studies conducted by contributors provide much practical advice for beginners as well as new ideas for experienced researchers. Some authors take a formal approach, but others speak quite personally in the first person. We hope you catch their enthusiasm and have fun conducting your own studies.

Mary de Chesnay

Acknowledgments

In any publishing venture, there are many people who work together to produce the final draft. The contributors kindly shared their expertise to offer advice and counsel to novices, and the reviewers ensured the quality of submissions. All of them have come up through the ranks as qualitative researchers and their participation is critical to helping novices learn the process.

No publication is successful without great people who not only know how to do their own jobs but also how to guide authors. At Springer Publishing Company, we are indebted to Margaret Zuccarini for the idea for the series, her ongoing support, and her excellent problem-solving skills. The person who guided the editorial process and was available for numerous questions, which he patiently answered as if he had not heard them a hundred times, was Joseph Morita. Also critical to the project were the people who proofed the work, marketed the series, and transformed it to hard copies, among them Jenna Vaccaro and Kris Parrish.

At Kennesaw State University, Dr. Tommie Nelms, director of the WellStar School of Nursing, was a constant source of emotional and practical support in addition to her chapter contribution to the phenomenology volume. Her administrative assistant, Mrs. Cynthia Elery, kindly assigned student assistants to complete several chores, which enabled the author to focus on the scholarship. Bradley Garner, Chadwick Brown, and Chino Duke are our student assistants and unsung heroes of the university.

Finally, I am grateful to my cousin, Amy Dagit, whose expertise in proofreading saved many hours for some of the chapters. Any mistakes left are mine alone.

> A people without the knowledge of their past history, origin, and culture is like a tree without roots.
>
> —Marcus Garvey

CHAPTER ONE

LEARNING THE HISTORICAL METHOD: STEP BY STEP

Sandra B. Lewenson and Annemarie McAllister

No occupation can be understood or intelligently followed if it is not, to some extent, illumined by the light of history.
—Stewart & Austin, 1962, p. 3

There are many ways to do historical research. Yet, getting started is the most difficult step, especially if you have not had formal training in the historical method. If you are not in an environment with a cadre of historians, especially nurse historians, or historians whose interest is in women's work, nursing, and health care, you can be at a disadvantage in learning this method and can feel discouraged. Yet many in nursing overcome these deficits and become scholars in the historical method and historical content of nursing. They do so by taking courses in history and historical methods, attending history conferences, participating in workshops on methodology, networking with other historians, and essentially learning the method through the experience of doing studies. Nurse historians are nurses who have studied the historical method and bring to their research the added dimension of a nursing background. One's experiences as a nurse contribute to the questions formed during the research process. They lead the scientist to examine data like nurses' role in public health nursing or in the movement toward higher education in nursing. For example, drawing on her own nursing background, Annemarie McAllister, a nurse historian, had firsthand experience at being an associate degree nurse in the 1970s through attending one of the early programs in the United States designed by Mildred Montag. As McAllister (2012) designed her doctoral research, she read through the materials and kept raising the question: "How did Montag and McManus change the face of nursing education so quickly?" Nursing was typically slow to change, especially when it came to moving nursing education outside of the hospital-based setting. While other historians might address the data similarly, they might not have the same insights that a nurse historian, like McAllister, may have. It is important to note here that biases, stereotypes, and other subjective responses of either the nurse historian or the historian who studies nursing may seep into the study and, while not fatal, should be recognized as offering one point of view rather than the "definitive" point of view.

This first chapter in this series explores the value of historical research, especially in nursing and health care; it covers the steps necessary for doing this kind of research and provides reasons why the researcher would select this method. The steps in becoming a historian are not linear and are described here as steps only to help delineate parts of a larger process of becoming a historical researcher. This chapter explores what is necessary when approaching this method, the steps that lead you through the process, and considerations that need to be addressed as you journey through the historical method. This chapter will also serve as a guide for Chapter 3, where Annemarie McAllister presents her experiences about becoming a historian during her doctoral work at Teachers College (TC), Columbia University.

VALUE OF HISTORICAL RESEARCH

Nursing leaders have long been aware of the need to understand the profession's history as a means to know the past, sort out the present, and direct the future. In the over 100 years since the beginning of what's known as the modern nursing movement, beginning when Florence Nightingale influenced the opening of training schools in the United States in 1873, early 20th century nursing leaders like Adelaide Nutting, Isabel Stewart, Lavinia Dock, and others recognized and spoke about the value of historical knowledge. The National League of Nursing Education, an early professional nursing organization established in 1896 by the superintendents of the early training schools, published curriculum guides in 1917, 1927, and 1937 respectively; these guides included content on the value of nursing history as well as content related to this relevant method. By the 1970s, however, most schools no longer included a separate course in nursing history; this may have been due to the decreasing value placed on history by nurses. Ultimately, this hindered the development of nurse researchers interested in doing historical research.

During the 1960s and 1970s resurgence in historical research, social histories, specifically those looking at nurses and women's work, found nurses interested in this particular method of inquiry (Lewenson, 2013a). Lucille

Notter, the editor of early editions of *Nursing Research*, believed that nurses, especially nursing leaders, needed to understand history as well as know the method in order to bring a broad perspective to the profession (Christy, 1978). Despite this renewed interest in doing historical research, some within nursing, in general, and among educators, more specifically, resisted the movement. This resistance stemmed partly from ignorance of the method and partly from what they perceived as lack of scholarly rigor in historical research. Quantitative research served as the gold standard for nursing leaders, who sought scientific parity and respect from other professions. Christy (1978) highlighted this in her presentation at the 1977 Isabel Stewart Nursing Research Conference at TC, Columbia. She said that nurses have disdained historical research because they consider it to be more "search than research," assuming it is *easy* and lacking rigor. Yet, Christy implored, "nothing can be further from the truth" (p. 5).

Nurse historians like Theresa Christy, Vern and Bonnie Bullough, Nettie Birnbach, Louise Fitzpatrick, Joan Lynaugh, Barbara Brodie, and many others expanded on the method using a social, feminist, and more progressive focus when studying nursing's past. The resurgence in the study of nursing history became even more apparent in the organization of the Society for Nursing History at TC and Boston's Nursing Archives Association; these predated the start of the American Association for the History of Nursing (AAHN), which was founded in 1978 (AAHN, 2013; Lewenson, 2013a; Lynaugh, 2009). The AAHN began as an organization for those studying historical research methodology and has continued to expand its interest in the promotion of historical research. Its website (AAHN, 2013) states its purpose—fostering the importance of history by stimulating interest, educating nurses, supporting research, facilitating collections of documents, serving as a resource, and promoting collaboration.

Throughout the world, the establishment of organizations such as the Canadian Association for the History of Nursing (CAHN), the Australian Nursing History & Midwifery Project, the British Columbia History of Nursing Group, and the Danish Society of Nursing History added to the support for historians as they matured in using this scholarly method of inquiry (Lewenson, 2013a). Increasing global attention to explore nursing in a broader global context has become evident in international conferences like the one held at the Royal Holloway College in Egham in 2010. This conference was sponsored by the AAHN along with the European Nursing History Group (ENHG) consisting of the UK Centre for the History of Nursing and Midwifery; the Irish Centre for Nursing and Midwifery History; Kingston University, London; St. George's, University of London; and the Royal College of Nursing History and Heritage Committee. History sections at the International Council of Nursing and Sigma Theta Tau also testify to the increasing relevance and value attributed to this kind of research (Lewenson, 2013a). The most recent work by D'Antonio, Fairman, and Whelan (2013), *Routledge Handbook on the Global History of Nursing*, presents the work of scholars who "consider new understandings of the historical work and worth of nursing in a larger global context" (p. 2).

Yet, as nurse historian Joan Lynaugh pointed out in an address presented at the Randolph International Nursing History Conference at the University of Virginia on March 20, 2009, while we are making progress in explaining the value of nursing history to fellow nursing colleagues, it is "still easier to explain nursing to our history colleagues" (Lynaugh, 2009, p. 14). Value and recognition for the history of nursing must start somewhere. The AAHN supports the inclusion of history in all nursing curricula (Keeling, 2001; Keeling & Ramos, 1995; Lewenson, 2004). Keeling believes that incorporating history and historical methodology into nursing curricula will "expand students' thinking," provide them with a "sense of professional heritage and identity," and "broaden the students' repertoire of research skills" (Keeling, 2001, para. 5). Without the inclusion of history in the curriculum and appreciation for its value to nurses in practice, education, and research, opportunities for the development and mentoring of new historians are limited.

Why Select the Method?

Following an understanding of the value of nursing history, the next step in the process of becoming a historian is to consider your own reasons for selecting the historical method. Your interest and the research question should direct the method that you will use to study your topic. Historical research provides the depth and breadth of what may have gone on before, allowing the researcher to view the topic within a contextual framework. The historian Christopher Maggs (1996) explains that, "the historian sees a multiplicity of events, facts, acts, and tries to reconstruct not just what happened but why it did so in the way and form it did" (p. 631). Historical analysis provides nurses with a way of knowing about their profession such as how it fits within the larger context of health care and medical advancement, how it may have influenced health care policy, or how issues related to gender, race, and ethnicity intersect with the economics and politics of care. For example, Keeling and Lewenson (2013) use their historical research to educate nurses and policy makers about the role nurses have historically played, and still play, in promoting and providing access to primary health care. They use as case studies the history of three nurse-run community services established during the first half of the 20th century that provided primary health care to underserved populations in urban and rural settings. The first one is the Henry Street Nurses' Settlement House on the Lower East Side of New York City, established by public health nursing leader Lillian Wald in 1893; the second example is the establishment of a rural public health nursing service by the American Red Cross that existed from 1912 to 1948; and the third is the Frontier Nursing Service that served the rural citizens of Leslie County, Kentucky, between 1920 and 1950 (Keeling & Lewenson, 2013). Keeling and Lewenson used these three examples to show nursing's leadership in bringing care to underserved populations and by employing interdisciplinary models to do so. They believe that the current debate about medical homes and who should lead the care provided by these homes is served by historical inquiry. Keeling and Lewenson, both nurse historians interested in public health, access to care, and policy issues, show the connection between these three historical nursing organizations and decisions being made today, specifically with regard to decisions being made about medical homes. Policy makers who are developing the federal policies surrounding medical homes, they believe, need to be aware of nursing's past contributions as well as the contributions they make today and will make in the future. Keeling and Lewenson (2013) write:

> Time and time again, nurses have demonstrated the expertise and experience that *makes* ... them poised to be valuable partners and leaders of the new developing models. Federal funding is necessary to support both nursing education and nursing practice initiatives as well as interprofessional models rather than a medical home model led only by physicians. What is needed is a unified interprofessional comprehensive service that includes, among others, nurses as leaders. The new model should therefore use neutral provider language. It behoves health policy makers to examine what was successful in the past and what needs to be changed to adapt to the present social, political, and economic health care environment. (n.p.)

The reason to select the historical method should be based on what the researcher hopes to do. To uncover what happened in the past is important; however, perhaps more important is to consider what and how this data will inform something that is current. Continuing with the example of how history can inform policy, D'Antonio and Fairman (2010) explain that, "history provides a critically important perspective if we are to understand and address contemporary health system problems ... [and] ... History also provides a way to look forward" (p. 113).

Although other chapters in this monograph address the state of the art of historical research in nursing, publications highlighting historical research will showcase the interests of historians as they make sense of the health care environment today. Examples of some of the research published include Arlene Keeling's (2007) work titled *Nursing and the Privilege of Prescription, 1893–2000*, where she examines nurses' use of medications in their practice; Patricia D'Antonio's (2010) work *American Nursing: A History of Knowledge, Authority and the Meaning of Work*; Julie Fairman's (2008) work exploring the history of the nurse practitioner movement in the United States, *Making Room in the Clinic: Nurse Practitioners and the Evolution of Modern Health Care*; Cynthia Connolly's (2008) book, *Saving Sickly Children: The Tuberculosis Preventorium in American Life, 1909–1970*, which uses the care provided to children who were at risk of developing tuberculosis to help us understand how we care for childhood epidemics today. Connolly's interest in pediatrics, policy, and politics, as well as the intersection of race, class, and gender, can be seen in her work. Edited texts, like the one by Patricia D'Antonio and Sandra Lewenson (2011), *Nursing Interventions Through Time: History as Evidence*, showcase their own interest in using historical research to understand contemporary nursing care. They include research by historians who examine the changing nursing interventions for bedsores, cancer, and obstetrics, for example, to demonstrate the interplay of gender, race, and class and the kind of care provided. In Barbra Mann Wall and Arlene Keeling's work (2011), *Nurses on the Front Line: When Disaster Strikes 1870–2010*, Wall and Keeling's own interest in history, and how communities address disaster, prompted the collection of their own research and the research of other historians.

Trends in more recent historical research places nursing within the larger context of the world-at-large and can be seen in the work by D'Antonio and colleagues (2013). The meanings that can be obtained through historical research impact nursing in other countries, the politics of care, and the effect of nationalism, colonialism, and war, for example, on that care. The editors write, "The history of nurses and nursing is now mined for insights that help explain or illustrate the global circulation [of] ideas about the care of the sick; about gender and valuation of care work; about the intersections of lay and professional care; and about the definitions and valuations of vulnerable populations" (p. 2). Lewenson's (2013a) chapter, "Historical Research in Nursing: A Current Outlook," included in Cheryl Tatono Beck's (2013) *Routledge International Handbook of Qualitative Nursing Research*, provides further examples of how historical research gives evidence for practice, education, and research and lays out a broad understanding of the state of historical research today.[1]

STEPS OF HISTORICAL RESEARCH

Table 1.1 *Steps in Doing Historical Research*

- Identify area of interest
- Raise questions
- Formulate title
- Conduct literature review
- Interpret data
- Tell the story

Adapted from Lewenson (2008, 2011) and found in *Capturing Nursing History*, Chapter 3, p. 26.

What Is Your Interest?

There are many ways to approach historical research (Lewenson, 2008). The different frameworks—social, feminist, policy, biographical, or economic—can shape the way the historical study develops. Each of these types of frameworks helps the researcher develop questions and explore the phenomenon under study. For example, in McAllister's work (see Chapter 3 for a full discussion), she selected a social/educational framework examining the development of the associate degree model for the education of nurses in the 1950s. Her interest in the topic emerged from her own background in nursing and exposure to the history of nursing at TC. Questions arose about how the leadership at TC promoted the rise of this unique and innovative mid-20th century educational model within a very short time frame (9 years) (Montag, 1959). Using the doctoral coursework in the executive program for nurses at TC, McAllister explored each assignment from a historical perspective. This set the stage for her to explore the history of nursing education, specifically at TC, considered by many the mecca for graduate education of nurses throughout most of the 20th century. Issues, such as the nursing shortage at the end of World War II, provided important background data that led to the search for quicker and more economical ways to educate nurses. Research in nursing was taking on greater significance in the profession, and in 1953 the Institute of Research and Service in Nursing Education was established by R. Louise McManus, Director of the Department of Nursing Education at TC, along with others (McAllister, 2012). This was in keeping with the overall nursing profession's growing interest in research. McAllister completed several papers assigned to her in various doctoral courses, which supported her exploration into history. One such paper responded to the question, "What does the literature say about the need for your historical study?" and, "What is the rationale for using a historical approach to your problem?" This allowed McAllister to explore in depth why she was going to do historical research for her doctoral dissertation and directed her to examine the literature that would support the reasons for her decision to study R. Louise McManus, Mildred Montag, and the leadership at TC.

The first step in historical research then was really to explore McAllister's interests in greater depth and breadth; this led her to develop an understanding of the context of the time frame in question, which then led to the development of further questions that she posed to historical data. Historical research seeks to understand phenomenon that occurred in the past and as such cannot be done in a simple linear fashion. While a timeline will help the researcher organize the data collected during these various steps in the process, it is the questions that are raised about the event, the context in which the event occurred, and the meanings behind the event that lead to the narrowing of the topic and more focused questions as the process evolves.

What Are Your Questions?

One of McAllister's other advisors on the doctoral dissertation committee said that there are no answers, only more questions. This holds true for most research designs and especially the historical method. The ambiguity that historians often express about the method stems from this lack of clarity and incomplete, missing, or confounding data. Yet the questions direct the researcher regarding where and what to study. Questions help one keep an open mind and can lead the researcher in surprising directions that he or she had not considered earlier (Lewenson, 2008). Lynaugh (2009) asks that historians move away from "ideology, theory, or predetermined thesis," letting a set of open questions guide the research. These questions include: "What happened?" "When did it happen?" "What difference did it make?" and "Why should we care?" (Lynaugh, 2009, p. 16).

As you proceed in your historical study, keep an open mind. This will allow you to pose more questions and direct and redirect the study as you reflect on who you are, select additional readings, complete grant applications, submit your research to your institutional review board for approval, and determine the rationale and the purpose of the study. The research question focuses the study. By isolating some part of the topic, your study usually becomes more manageable. Yet, you as a researcher need to be aware of this split so that you can then ultimately relate to the whole in the analysis and answer the important questions of "So what?" and "Who cares?" These questions must be raised to make sense of why your work is relevant and meaningful to a larger audience. The audience you write for will also influence the questions you may ask. For example, consider an audience who is interested in celebrating the first 100 years of their school's history. This group may be more interested in the celebratory nature of their history rather than a critique of their educational experiences in comparison with another school. Your doctoral dissertation committee will be looking at the depth and breadth of your study, including such areas as your methodology, data collection, the frameworks you select, your analysis, and the narrative.

Determining a Title

How you name your study will be important for a number of reasons. First, it directs both you (the researcher) and the reader as to what the study is about. A clear and concise title will help readers or potential readers determine if they want to read your work. This includes reviewers for journals and conferences—a title that is interesting and captures the reader's imagination is more effective in enticing the reader. Second, a title may keep you focused; covering topics that don't relate to the title lets you know you have strayed from your plan. The title typically includes a succinct statement about the study, delineating the topic and the years being studied (Lewenson, 2008, 2011). It will not be easy to determine the title (or at least it was not easy for this researcher). The title needs to be concise, clear, and—perhaps more importantly—easy to search on web browsers. If you want to use a web-based search to find your study, include in the first part of your title sufficient information so that your study will be searchable. Consider the "Googled" findings for a study titled, "When One Door Opens Another Closes" versus "The Phasing out of the Bellevue and Mills Training Schools and the Expansion of Hunter College, 1967." The latter renders hits on Bellevue and Hunter College's two programs in nursing while the former renders nothing on the topic. Finding a title for any study can be challenging and very often changes throughout the process. For this reason, it may be best to finesse the final title at the end of the process. Another point to note when determining your title is that titles can change when the focus of the study changes, or when findings lead you in a different direction. For example, using the previous example, when studying the phasing out of the Bellevue and Mills Training Schools of Nursing and the expansion of Hunter College into the Bellevue facility in 1967, one title depicted this long explanation of phasing out and expansion and was used for presentations and explanations of the study; while reexamining the data focusing on the political ramifications of support from the City of New York for this change in nursing education, the author created a new title for the study. The new title, seemingly more catchy, used a quote from a newspaper clipping from 1967 that heralded the change in nursing education in the city with the phrase, "Nurses' training may be shifted." The study was published in *Nursing History Review* in 2013 with the title, "'Nurses' Training May Be Shifted': The Story of Bellevue and Hunter College, 1942–1969" (Lewenson, 2013b). Whether this captures more hits on a Google search is yet to be determined, but it seems to this author to be a more interesting title. The balance among what is interesting, catchy, encapsulating the essence of the study, and enticing is difficult to attain. Sharing your study with others to read, doing your own web searches for what shows up with your topic, and thinking about the title (almost ad nauseam) may help with finding the right one for the study. Run your proposed title by colleagues, friends, your advisor, and family and see what they say. As you struggle with naming your research, remember that, even though a title helps focus a new researcher (as well as a seasoned one), it should not restrict or limit the study that is underway.

Searching the Literature

The literature search continues throughout the historical research process. In other words, you start out reading materials that provide the contextual background and continue to read throughout the study, beginning with your interest in a particular topic, through the identification of background materials, the questions raised, the analysis, and the writing of the narrative (Lewenson, 2008). This is where the various types of source materials, both primary and secondary sources, become relevant in the steps along the way.

Secondary Sources

Secondary sources include materials that provide background for a specific period of time, a particular intervention, or a newspaper account of an event. Secondhand knowledge transmits a contextual backdrop to the topic under study. Many of the books mentioned earlier in this chapter are secondary sources. Fairman's (2008) analysis of the nurse practitioner movement, for example, is a secondary source that historians use to contextualize and understand the nurse practitioner movement in the United States during the second half of the 20th century. Secondary sources broaden the historian's understanding of a particular place or event and help the researcher to refocus and question the data. It is an ongoing part of the process, and one that perhaps will make the historian question, "When is enough, enough?" When do you stop reading, and, more importantly, when do you stop questioning? Both questions can be answered as both "never" and "at some point." These questions surface throughout the historian's foray into this type of research and are worth considering (these are discussed in a later section, and McAllister considers them in Chapter 3). While you may never really stop reading and questioning, you will need to do so (to some degree) to complete your dissertation or study in a reasonable amount of time. What can help here is to read other historical studies as guides for formats, frameworks, or writing styles; select a framework that will help focus your work, whether using a social–feminist framework, an economic framework, or a political framework; this will help you select reading that may help contextualize your findings (Buck, 2008).

Primary Sources

An important point for all those embarking on historical research is to consider the availability of primary source materials. A significant part of the search of the literature is locating primary source materials. Primary source materials offer firsthand accounts of an event or subject of interest. They can take the form of personal letters, diaries, organizational minutes, or financial ledgers lending insights into a particular place, time, person, or event. Because of the firsthand nature of primary sources, these documents may be subject to the personal bias of the author and should be considered a possible limitation of the study. For example, Mansell (1999) considers organizational minutes as perhaps being too one-sided when presenting a broader picture of nursing. It represents the events of organized nursing rather than the rank and file, thus limiting "the response to the research questions about 'class, status, and ethnicity' of these nurses as opposed to the leadership in nursing" (p. 220). Because primary sources may provide only one perspective, researchers must consider this in their analysis. McAllister's work, for example, observed that the records located at TC archives shed light mostly on what the educators involved in the establishment of the associate degree model considered important to retain in the official records. The records of those opposing the associate degree model, or perhaps the influence of TC on the landscape of nursing practice and education, were not included and were difficult to locate in other collections. Part of the work of the historian is to consider what kinds of primary materials exist, determine where they may be found, and analyze them in light of the framework (e.g., social, political, economic, feminist), the context in which the primary sources reside, the researcher's own bias that frames the way he or she considers the data (including the missing data), and the genuineness and authenticity of the source material (Lewenson, 2011). Genuineness refers to the document being what it says it is, and authenticity refers to whether the data found on that document make sense in light of the period of time to which it refers. For example, the researcher needs to ask if the document represents a truthful reporting of that period of time (Barzun & Graff, 1985).

Ensuring the integrity of the primary source material is not an easy task for the historian, and it is an especially challenging one for the novice. Archives, where historians typically find the primary sources (although not always), can help with the task of authenticating the source material. According to Barzun and Graff (1985), a researcher who is lucky enough to have found a stash of letters about his or her mother's experiences as a nurse during an earlier period of time may need to pay special attention to the details within the letters, common-sense reasoning, understanding of human behavior, and the chronology of events.

Where to Find Primary Sources

The primary source materials can typically be found in archives, like the ones located at the Bellevue Alumnae Center for Nursing in Guilderland, New York (www.foundationnysnurses.org/bellevue/index.php); the Barbara Bates Center for the Study of Nursing located at the University of Pennsylvania in Philadelphia (www.nursing.upenn.edu/history/Pages/default.aspx); or the Eleanor Crowder Bjoring Center for Nursing Historical Inquiry at the University of Virginia in Charlottesville, Virginia (www.nursing.virginia.edu/research/cnhi). These three archives provide rich data in which to study nurses and nursing history. The AAHN website (www.aahn.org) offers a comprehensive listing of other archives throughout the United States and globally, offering great opportunities for researchers who are pursuing a particular area in history. Archives differ from libraries in the kinds of documents stored, the way they are stored, the way they are used, the way they are identified, and the way they are documented. Archives use finders' guides to document their holdings, which are quite commonly posted on their website. Most archives require researchers to contact them directly to discuss the research they are doing, the kinds of documents that may exist in the collections, and the kinds of access a researcher may have to those collections. For example, most (if not all) archives require that the researcher make an appointment and visit the archives; in others, depending on the topic and amount of content that is available, the archivists might make copies to send to the researcher and save the researcher the expense of traveling to those archives (Lewenson, 2011).

Oral Histories

Oral histories serve as important primary source materials and can add depth and breadth to historical research. The topic and the period of time under study will determine whether or not one can collect oral histories. Topics that are situated within the mid- to late 20th century may still have some witnesses to events from that period of time. Interviewing nurses who knew Mildred Montag and R. Louise McManus, as in McAllister's study, provides insight into the personalities of these two leaders that could not be obtained from written documentation. Boschma, Scaia, Bonifacio, and Roberts (2008) explain that oral history gives "the narrator the freedom to express ideas and thoughts in a way that may not otherwise be preserved in a written form and about subjects that have not traditionally been topics of historical investigation" (p. 79). Oral histories offer firsthand accounts of a particular event in time; yet, like other source material, they contain the bias of that person's account of the event. The relationship between the interviewer, the interviewee, and the environment in which the event happens influences the story that emerges and must be accounted for by the historian in the final analysis and the written narration of that history.[2]

Interpret the Data

When completing oral histories for one of her own studies about the phasing out of Bellevue and Mills School of Nursing and the expansion of Hunter College Department of Nursing (Lewenson, 2013b) into that facility, McAllister used oral histories of students and alumnae from both schools to share their insights into what they experienced at the time of this change. Conflicting memories about how they learned of the change in schools or how they reacted to this event added dimension to the study that the written documentation by itself could not provide. McAllister's own perception, as someone who had also attended Hunter College at this same point of time, certainly added to the challenge of analyzing the data. Analysis included the placement of the themes that emerged from the oral histories in context with themes that emerged from the other primary source documents such as the minutes of the board of trustees, faculty notices, and city records. Interpretation of the data, placing it within a context of time and space, and framing the data—using the framework that you select, in this case a sociopolitical one—helps the researcher understand and explain in the narration or the telling of the story. The final step in the research process—narration—blends these themes together; in McAllister's study, it created a rich story reflecting how New York City balanced its financial concerns with those of higher education and health care in municipal-run organizations, as well as with the search for educational excellence at the Bellevue and Mills School of Nursing and Hunter College Department of Nursing, and with the personal and professional stories of individuals engaged in this educational change at both the leadership and the student level (Lewenson, 2013b).

Tell the Story

One of McAllister's favorite histories is the one by Elizabeth M. Norman (1999), *We Band of Angels: The Untold Story of American Nurses Trapped on Bataan by the Japanese*. Her prose reads like a novel, yet it is still a well-documented historical research work. Telling the story means pulling all the parts of your research together in a meaningful way that presents your findings in a coherent and organized manner that is also interesting to read. This is not easy and is a skill that requires practice and time to acquire. Narrating involves making sense of the data you have collected, responding to your questions, interpreting these findings for the audience, and making the history resonate with the reader. Comfort with the written word helps with coherently weaving the various parts together. It is a big job and one that requires the researcher to be creative. Nurse historian Joan Lynaugh (2000) explains that the challenge of writing the narrative means setting the time accurately, organizing the facts in the context of the period, and keeping the reader engaged and clinging to the story.

Other Considerations Along the Way

As the researcher progresses through the steps of historical research, other considerations need to be addressed. Issues that the researcher may face include ethical concerns related to the study and the submission of an institutional review board application; the cost to complete the study and grant opportunities to cover those costs; time constraints and the selection of advisors; and support of all kinds that will help expedite the work.

Ethical Concerns

Historical research requires the researcher to act ethically, honestly, and truthfully. Just as in other forms of research, historians experience ethical concerns such as how to handle data that may be sensational in nature or possibly harmful to the participants involved. While doing oral histories, consent forms must be obtained to protect the rights of the participants. These forms should include information about what can be published, and where it can be published. Other issues may arise when using photographs, which historians typically use in presentations and scholarly works. Are the photographs found on the Internet, or are they from an archive requiring a fee and acknowledgment? How does the historian use them—in scholarly presentations or in publications—and what kinds of permissions (and perhaps fees) are required when using these photographs? Lewenson and Herrmann (2008) refer historians to the *Ethical Guidelines for the Nurse Historian* and *Standards of Professional Conduct for Historical Inquiry in Nursing* developed by nurse historians Nettie Birnbach, Janie Brown, and Wanda Hiestand (Birnbach, 2008). Historians can refer to these two documents for questions about ethical behavior as they provide relevant talking points about what makes sense and what is expected. The responsibility of the historian to the primary and secondary sources, the subjects, students, community, and history can be found in the *Ethical Guidelines*. According to this document, some of the responsibilities a historian undertakes during the research process include sharing knowledge, mentoring others, advocating the preservation of historic documents, and expecting to be true to the data (Birnbach, 2008). The second document, *The Standards of Professional Conduct*, outlines some of the responsibilities that historians assume during the process. These responsibilities are to the public, colleagues, students, subjects, research, and ethical canons of research. Some of the responsibilities that lay the groundwork for ethical discussions and behavior include acknowledging the work of others, engaging in peer review activities, including student participation in research projects, recognizing the value of historical research, and following the canons of historical inquiry (e.g., do not damage archival materials). The reader is encouraged to read both Birnbach's (2008) chapter "Ethical Guidelines and Standards of Professional Conduct" and Lewenson and Herrmann's (2008) chapter, "Using Ethical Guidelines and Standards of Professional Conduct," for a more complete discussion.

Institutional Review Board (IRB) Application

Most institutions require that the researcher undergo a review by an institutional review board (IRB). In this way, the rights of the participants and any ethical issues related to the method are considered and addressed at the outset of any research project. Locally based IRBs bear the responsibility of approving the "ethical acceptability" of a proposed research project, and the question of what kinds of research bear review vary depending on the funding sources being sought and federal requirements (American Association of University Professors [AAUP], 2013; Shopes, n.d.; Shopes, 2007). Although oral histories are not required by federal law to undergo the scrutiny of an IRB, many IRBs require the researcher to submit an application for the IRB to determine whether a review is needed or not. Because of the complicated and tenuous nature of determining the need for an IRB, Shopes (n.d.) recommends the following "reasonable course of action" for college or university students, scholars, or staff members undergoing an oral history project:

1. Inform yourself of the federal regulations.
2. Seek allies within your department or relevant administrative unit.
3. Take a proactive approach with the IRB, informing it of the principles and practices governing history in general and oral history in particular and insisting that it conform to the federal requirement that an IRB include or consult with individuals who can knowledgeably review any proposed research, in this case an individual with adequate knowledge of oral history.
4. Provide a forum for discussing "real ethics" in oral history. (Shopes, n.d., para. starting with "What to Do")

Typically, historical research, whether inclusive of oral history or not, undergoes an expedited institutional review, which still requires the researcher to respond to questions assuring the protection of participants. The historian needs to be able to prepare the documentation required by the IRB and include any letters of consent for oral histories and other documentation regarding the use of the data in the study. Those completing oral histories should follow the oral history association's (OHA) *Principles and Best Practices for Oral History*, which includes what historians need to follow (OHA, 2009). Consent forms signed by oral history participants must be included in the IRB application and should be part of the study regardless of whether the IRB requires it or not. The letter should include information about the study, ownership of the copyright of the data, where the transcripts will be stored following the study, and the rights of the narrator (the person being interviewed). The consent can be signed or recorded prior to the collection of data (OHA, 2009).

Covering Costs

Aside from the ethical and methodological issues one faces, covering the cost of historical research is a huge consideration. While grant money is available, few fund historical research. Whelan and Connolly (2008) advocate applying for grant money for several reasons including obtaining financial resources, and, perhaps equally important, for "currency in the scholarly world" (p. 181). These authors write that obtaining external funding for a historian "is a recognized credential that reinforces the notion that historical research is knowledge-generative research and not 'fun nostalgia'" (p. 181). It is important to note here that the AAHN has several external grant opportunities available to nurse historians. In addition, the various history centers mentioned earlier in this chapter offer funding opportunities as well (check the AAHN.org website for a listing of additional grant opportunities).

Possible costs that you need to consider include the purchase of books and materials to enhance the ease of research; travel to archival collections, which includes such expenses as transportation, hotel, and meals; purchases of electronic equipment to help with the collection and organization of data (although free downloads for the organizing Zotero—www.zotero.org—help; in addition, laptops, digital cameras, and smartphones will help with the collection of data at various archives and libraries and will be essential when collecting oral histories); transcription costs for oral histories; photocopies for primary source material (although you can use your camera or smartphone to photograph documents if the archives permit its use; if so, be sure to include the identifying data on the photograph so that you will know where you found it if you decide to use the data in your study); membership in history organizations (e.g., AAHN); and attendance at professional meetings that can enhance your understanding of the method as well as the content of your study (thus requiring consideration for registration costs, hotel, and food). Since other costs may also arise, determining ways to cut costs will be helpful—for example, identifying primary sources that you can travel to at a reasonable expense. If you have identified primary sources located at a great distance and cost, check with the archives first to see if they have what you are looking for or if there is any way materials can be photocopied or electronically sent to you before you make your trip.

Time Constraints

For all researchers, time is important. For those going through the doctoral process, the process can be overwhelming. Completing a dissertation in a timely fashion that allows one to graduate not too far from completing the coursework is the goal. Yet, historical research takes time. Reading, identifying your interest, selecting the historical method (and then learning the method if unfamiliar with it), selecting advisors and mentors who can expedite the process (rather than slow it down as in some cases), locating the primary and secondary sources, traveling to the archives, addressing ethical and financial issues, applying for funding, completing oral histories, and writing the narrative all contribute to completing the study in a "reasonable" amount of time. Although there is no set reasonable amount of time for conducting research, as historian Nettie Birnbach stated to McAllister years ago, "it's not your life work—go home and work with what you have." As Birnback offered this advice, McAllister sat in the old *American Journal of Nursing* library in New York City where she had been reading through the many nursing journals from 1898 to 1920 for evidence connecting nurses and nursing to the women's movement during that same period. After being at this collection stage for over a year, McAllister had piles of materials stacked beside her, yet she continued to search (sometimes repeatedly search) for these kinds of references (this was before the digitalization of *AJNs* or any other journal of nursing). It was finally time to stop—McAllister was faced with what Fondiller (1978, p. 26) describes as "every researcher's fear of overlooking some splendid gem of historical import." Fondiller advised that at some point, one has to "work with what you have" (p. 26). Learning when to stop is crucial, especially when time is of the essence, meaning doctoral students should be graduating within a year or two of when they complete their coursework, assuming that they have worked throughout their coursework on parts of the research process.

The selection of one's doctoral committee advisor or a mentor for one's historical research is extremely important to the process as a whole and, in particular, to the time you will spend on your dissertation. Find advisors and mentors who are willing, have the expertise (whether in content or method), and have the time to help move you through the process. In other words, they need to be able to read your material in a timely fashion and be available to you when you need a response (or friendly voice). What is meant by "timely fashion" should be determined by both the advisee and advisor, and fit the expectations of both. While a quick turnaround time for a question or critique of a particular section of the dissertation is desired, especially by the student, it is not always possible for the faculty. The converse is true when the faculty expects work to be delivered, and the student is unable to do so at an agreed time. It's a dance, if you will. Both parties (and you are typically dealing with the schedules of several educators on the committee) must negotiate a timeline, a schedule of when and how material will be returned, when meetings will occur, and how often you will meet. Very often, meeting by phone, Skype, or Microsoft Lync (or some other electronic means of connecting) can offer solutions for long distance communication alleviating the time and expanse of traveling to the campus.

All research takes time; for novice historians, it may take even more time. Newton (1965) wrote that "Historical research leads the student down one path and another until he is amazed and must decide when to stop" (Newton, 1965, p. 25).

Next Steps

Once you have completed your study and have had it approved by your committee, you are ready to take the next step of dissemination. Throughout your dissertation, you need to submit the various sections as you go to different conferences (here is where networking with other nurse historians at the AAHN will be helpful as the organization holds a doctoral luncheon at every annual meeting where doctoral students from all over meet to share with others) and consider where and what parts of your dissertation you will be submitting for publication. These next steps are all part of the journey of becoming a nurse historian and considering your next historical study. Although one never really stops reading and questioning (as noted earlier), you should be considering your next research project, building on what you have been doing in your first. Your advisors, mentors, and your colleagues in your program will help you through this whole process as well as help you discover what your next steps may be and where they will take you.

NOTES

1. The American Association for the History of Nursing (AAHN) website provides a more complete listing of published books, articles, and websites that will help a budding historian determine whether the historical method is the right design for his or her own interest in a topic.
2. For additional resources and a more in-depth discussion, see the Oral History Association website (www.oralhistory.org); also see Chapter 5 by Boschma in this book.

REFERENCES

American Association for the History of Nursing (AAHN). (2013). Retrieved from http://www.aahn.org/about.html

American Association of University Professors (AAUP). (2013, March). Regulation of research on human subjects: Academic freedom and the Institutional Review Board. Retrieved from http://www.oralhistory.org/wp-content/uploads/2013/03/IRB-Final-Report.pdf

Barzun, J., & Graff, H. F. (1985). *The modern researcher* (4th ed.). San Diego, CA: Harcourt Brace Jovanovich.

Birnbach, N. (2008). Ethical guidelines and standards of professional conduct. In S. B. Lewenson & E. K. Herrmann (Eds.), *Capturing nursing history: A guide to historical methods in research* (pp. 167–172). New York, NY: Springer Publishing.

Boschma, G., Scaia, M., Bonifacio, N., & Roberts, E. (2008). Oral history research. In S. B. Lewenson & E. K. Herrmann (Eds.), *Capturing nursing history: A guide to historical methods in research.* New York, NY: Springer Publishing.

Buck, J. (2008). Using frameworks in historical research. In S. B. Lewenson & E. K. Herrmann (Eds.), *Capturing nursing history: A guide to historical methods in nursing* (pp. 45–62). New York, NY: Springer Publishing.

Christy, T. (1978). The hope of history. In M. L. Fitzpatrick (Ed.), *Historical studies in nursing: Papers presented at the 15th annual Stewart Conference on research in nursing March 1977* (pp. 3–11). New York, NY: Teachers College Press.

Connolly, C. A. (2008). *Saving sickly children: The tuberculosis preventorium in American life, 1909–1970.* New Brunswick, NJ: Rutgers University Press.

D'Antonio, P. (2010). *American nursing: A history of knowledge, authority and the meaning of work.* Baltimore, MD: Johns Hopkins University Press.

D'Antonio, P., & Fairman, J. A. (2010). History matters. *Nursing Outlook, 58,* 113–114.

D'Antonio, P., Fairman, J. A., & Whelan, J. C. (Eds.). (2013). *Routledge handbook on the global history of nursing.* London, UK: Routledge, Taylor & Francis Group.

D'Antonio, P., & Lewenson, S. B. (Eds.). (2011). *Nursing interventions through time: History as evidence.* New York, NY: Springer Publishing.

Fairman, J. (2008). *Making room in the clinic: Nurse practitioners and the evolution of modern health care.* New Jersey, NJ: Rutgers Press.

Fondiller, S. (1978). Writing the report. In M. L. Fitzpatrick (Ed.), *Historical studies in nursing* (pp. 25–27). New York, NY: Teachers College Press.

Keeling, A. W. (2001). Nursing history in the curriculum: Preparing nurses for the 21st century. American Association for the History of Nursing (AAHN). Retrieved from http://www.aahn.org/about.html

Keeling, A. W. (2007). *Nursing and the privilege of prescription, 1893–2000.* Columbus, OH: Ohio State Press.

Keeling, A. W., & Lewenson, S. B. (2013). A nursing historical perspective on the medical home: Impact on health policy. *Nursing Outlook, 61*(5), 360–366.

Keeling, A. W., & Ramos, M. C. (1995). The role of nursing history in preparing nursing for the future. *Nursing and Health Care, 16*(l), 30–34.

Lewenson, S. B. (2004). Integrating nursing history in the curriculum. *Journal of Professional Nursing, 20*(6), 374–380.

Lewenson, S. B. (2008). Doing historical research. In S. B. Lewenson & E. K. Herrmann (Eds.), *Capturing nursing history: A guide to historical methods in research* (pp. 25–43). New York, NY: Springer Publishing.

Lewenson, S. B. (2011). Historical research method. In H. J. Speziale & D. R. Carpenter (Eds.), *Qualitative research in nursing: Advancing the humanistic imperative* (5th ed., pp. 225–248). Philadelphia, PA: Lippincott.

Lewenson, S. B. (2013a). Historical research in nursing: A current outlook. In C. T. Beck (Ed.), *Routledge international handbook of qualitative nursing research* (pp. 256–267). New York: Routledge.

Lewenson, S. B. (2013b). Nurses' training may be shifted: The story of Bellevue and Hunter College, 1942–1969. *Nursing History Review, 21,* 14–32.

Lewenson, S. B., & Herrmann, E. K. (2008). Using ethical guidelines and standards of professional conduct. In S. B. Lewenson & E. K. Herrmann (Eds.), *Capturing nursing history: A guide to historical methods in research* (pp. 173–179). New York, NY: Springer Publishing.

Lynaugh, J. E. (2000). Editorial. *Nursing History Review, 8.*

Lynaugh, J. (2009, May). *"In and out of favor": Scholarship and nursing history.* Keynote address presented at the Randolph International Nursing History Conference, Charlottesville, VA.

Maggs, C. (1996). A history of nursing: A history of caring? *Journal of Advanced Nursing, 23,* 630–635.

Mansell, D. (1999). Sources in nursing historical research: A thorny methodological problem. *Canadian Journal of Nursing Research, 30*(4), 219–222.

McAllister, A. (2012). *R. Louise McManus and Mildred Montag create the associate degree model for the education of nurses: The right leaders, the right time, the right place: 1947 to 1959.* Unpublished doctoral dissertation, Teachers College, Columbia University.

Montag, M. L. (1959). *Community college education for nursing: An experiment in technical education for nursing.* New York, NY: McGraw-Hill.

Newton, M. E. (1965). The case for historical research. *Nursing Research, 14*(1), 20–26.

Norman, E. (1999). *We Band of Angels: The Untold Story of American Nurses Trapped on Bataan by the Japanese.* New York: Simon & Schuster.

Oral History Association (OHA). (2009). *Principles and best practices principles for oral history and best practices for oral history association.* Retrieved from http://www.oralhistory.org/about/principles-and-practices

Shopes, L. (n.d.). Oral history, human subjects, and institutional review boards. *Oral history association.* Retrieved from http://www.oralhistory.org/about/do-oral-history/oral-history-and-irb-review/

Shopes, L. (2007). Forum on IRBs: Negotiating institutional review boards. *American Historical Association (AHA) Perspectives Online, 43*(3), n.p. Retrieved from http://www.historians.org/perspectives/issues/2007/0703/0703vie1.cfm

Stewart, I. M., & Austin, A. L. (1962). *A history of nursing from ancient to modern times: A world view* (5th ed.). New York, NY: G. P. Putnam's Sons.

Wall, B. M., & Keeling, A. W. (Eds.). (2011). *Nurses on the front line: When disaster strikes 1870–2010.* New York, NY: Springer Publishing.

Whelan, J. C., & Connolly, C. A. (2008). Funding for historical research. In S. B. Lewenson & E. K. Herrmann (Eds.), *Capturing nursing history: A guide to historical methods in research* (pp. 181–197). New York, NY: Springer Publishing.

CHAPTER TWO

ESSAY ON SOURCES

Patricia D'Antonio

As I think about the scholarship that has informed my approach to the history of nursing, I feel something like an archeologist systematically surveying the texts in my bookcases, excavating hidden gems that I have not thought about in quite some time, and articulating connections between the exemplary work of those who have come before me and my own interpretations. This essay is by no means exhaustive. Researchers writing about nursing's history from positions both within and outside the discipline have produced a rich body of studies about individuals, training schools and colleges, animating ideas, and actual practices. A survey of the articles published in the volumes of the *Nursing History Review*, the official journal of the American Association for the History of Nursing, and in *Nursing Inquiry* provides immediate access to the breadth and depth of this particular field of inquiry. Both journals provide a space where scholars from many different disciplines come together to explore the ways in which the histories of nurses and nursing intersect with those that explore the possibilities and the problems of fundamental human importance around the globe.

This essay, by contrast, allows me to acknowledge my personal intellectual debts. Like any good archeologist, then, I must return to the beginning: to M. Adelaide Nutting and Lavinia L. Dock's majestic, four-volume *A History of Nursing* (1907–1912). Nutting and Dock's explicit intent was to make visible what had been invisible. And their rationale still echoes in many of those proposed by historians of nursing today. They wanted to counter "long ages of silence" about gentler and more humane acts that made human

---

Editor's note: We are grateful to Johns Hopkins University Press for permission to reprint Dr. D'Antonio's work. D'Antonio, Patricia. *American nursing: A history of knowledge, authority, and the meaning of work*, pp. 231–243. © 2010 Johns Hopkins University Press. Reprinted with permission of Johns Hopkins University Press.

society possible; to challenge "...the tendency of historians to overlook what was usual and homely"; and to show nurses how their history was inexorably linked with that of other women. "As they rise," they wrote, "she rises, and as they sink, she falls" (Nutting & Dock, 1907, pp. 5, v).

The first two volumes, both published in 1907, take the reader on a stirring sweep of *The Evolution of Nursing Systems From the Earliest Times to the Foundation of the First English and American Training Schools for Nurses*. We travel from the care of preliterate peoples to that of ancient Greece and Rome. We track the care available in families to that in the rising religious orders. We dread the 18th century's "dark period" that coincided with the general subjugation of women. Yet we revel in the 19th century's revival presaged by the German deaconate and fulfilled in the triumphs of Florence Nightingale. Dock edited the last two volumes, *From Earliest Times to the Present Day With Special Reference to the Work of the Past Thirty Years*. Both were published in 1912, and both contained essays by nurses around the globe describing the emergence of trained nursing in their respective countries. These volumes take their readers on tours of nursing in Japan and China. They take them into leper colonies in the Philippines and into the Cama Hospital in Bombay. Most of the stories are of White nursing women sponsored by religious missions and colonial governments and charged with the care of indigenous peoples. But the reader sees hope for the future in proud pictures of small graduating classes of native-born women in such places as Syria, Korea, and Cuba.

There is much that we, with more modern eyes, might point to as wrong about Dock and Nutting's *A History of Nursing*. It is about great women doing great things within the great sweep of historical time. The authors themselves —Dock and Nutting and their various contributors—are blind to their privileges of race and class. Their enshrinement of the "trio of training schools" —those at the Bellevue Hospital in New York City, the New Haven Hospital in Connecticut, and the Massachusetts General Hospital in Boston—as those from which the steady march of nursing progress in America dates has long obscured the important role played by earlier nurses' training initiatives.

Yet, one cannot help but be moved by Dock and Nutting's passion, optimism, confidence, and intellect. They were the true children of their era: Progressives certain that the rational application of knowledge would lead to substantive change; educated women asserting their right to power and a public voice; and clinicians, like their medical colleagues at Johns Hopkins, seeking to harness their history in service to their newly articulated claims to scientific authority. Diane Hamilton, in "Constructing the Mind of Nursing," places these women in an early 20th century "thought collective" that intellectually reified compassion as one of the basic guiding principles of the new discipline (Hamilton, 1994). But, for me, their powerful narrative demanded that I take them, their ideas, their institutions, and their vision seriously. It also shaped how I came to look for and understand the ways in which nurses created and maintained a powerful and shared internal identity that served as a defense against social perceptions that often belied their sense of themselves. Not surprisingly, *A History of Nursing* was condensed into a one-volume text in 1920. The renamed *A Short History of Nursing* quickly became required reading for generations of nursing students (Dock & Stewart, 1920).

By midcentury, the pride of place held by *A History of Nursing* yielded to other authors and other perspectives. Some, like Victor Robinson in *White Caps: The Story of Nursing* (1946) and Richard Shyrock in *History of Nursing: An Interpretation of the Social and Medical Factors Involved* (1959), were constructed by physicians turning to the history of nursing after completing works on the history of medicine. Most, however, were by nurses looking toward nurses as their primary audience. Mary Roberts, then editor of the *American Journal of Nursing*, published *American Nursing: History and Interpretation* (1954) that, not surprisingly, focused on the place of leaders and leading institutions in the history of nursing. Josephine Dolan's varyingly titled histories of nursing held prominence from the 1960s through the 1980s.[1] These texts favored facts over interpretative leaps. But historians who tend toward more analytic work can often overlook the critical importance of factually accurate texts. The varying editions of texts by Philip A. Kalish and Beatrice J. Kalish have been particularly useful in my own work. I have depended heavily on the third edition of *The Advance of American Nursing* (1986).

But, at the same time these texts were rolling off publishers' presses, the field of nursing history was in the process of a profound transformation. If the triumphant *A History of Nursing* was the first book I read, Jo Ann Ashley's devastating *Hospitals, Paternalism and the Role of the Nurse* (1976) was the second. Ashley unfurled a furious—and controversial—critique of the sexism of male physicians and hospital administrators that had kept nurses subservient for generations. It was, like *A History of Nursing*, a work of passion. But unlike its early 20th century predecessor, Ashley's historical nurses were curiously passive and even complicit in their own subordination.

This theme of subordination runs through some of the more recent studies on the history of nursing. Mary Poovey's classic argument in *Uneven Developments: The Ideological Work of Gender in Mid-Victorian England* (1988) that nursing never realized its potentially subversive threat to gendered roles still carries weight. The Nightingale-inspired positioning of women nurses in a traditionally hierarchical ordering vis-à-vis male physicians, she argued, signaled an end to a battle over roles before it had even begun. Joan Roberts and Thetis Group's *Feminism and Nursing: An Historical Perspective on Power, Status, and Political Activism in the Nursing Profession* (1995) and their later *Nursing, Physician Control, and the Medical Monopoly* (2001) return to this theme but unfortunately with more of Ashley's stridency than Poovey's nuances. A more insightful iteration of the theme of subordination can be seen in the work of literary theorist Kristine Swenson, who borrows Poovey's methodological combination of historical and textural analysis. In *Medical Women and Victorian Fiction* (2005), Swenson's "New Woman" doctors emerge as more significant actors than nurses in shaping Britain's late 19th century medical practice because they more easily rejected the ideology of separate spheres of influence in the process of becoming emancipated professionals.

Florence Nightingale, of course, remains the lightning rod in these analyses. Few actors have captured historians' attention to the extent that she has. There seems to be a biography that matches whatever one's mood. If one feels quietly congratulatory, read Cecil Woodham-Smith's well-regarded *Florence Nightingale, 1820–1910* (1950). If one feels rather cross about her influence, turn to F. B. Smith's manipulative and self-aggrandizing villain in *Florence Nightingale: Reputation and Power* (1982). And if one is feeling rather pressed for time, pick up a remarkable yet underrated collection of essays in Vern Bullough, Bonnie Bullough, and Marietta Stanton's *Florence Nightingale and Her Era: A Collection of New Scholarship* (1990).

More recently, researchers have tended to focus on particular moments in Nightingale's life. Hugh Small's *Florence Nightingale: Avenging Angel* (1999) focuses on her time in the Crimea and her deep distress when she discovered that the mortality rates at her own hospital in Scutari were higher than those at British hospitals elsewhere in the region. Monica Baly's *Florence Nightingale and the Nursing Legacy* (1997) turns to the famous nurses' training school at St. Thomas' in London and suggests that much of its success came from a well-oiled publicity machine. Jharna Gourlay's *Florence Nightingale and the Health of the Raj* (2003) focuses on Nightingale's involvement with India and charts her movement from a narrow focus only on the health of the British Army to a much broader perspective that supported political changes as a means to address the subcontinent's social and economic concerns. Gillian Gill's *Nightingales: The Extraordinary Upbringing and Curious Life of Miss Florence Nightingale* (2004) returns to Nightingale's childhood and suggests that, far from being an enigma to a staunchly bourgeois family, Nightingale grew up surrounded by a warm circle of intellectually curious, socially committed, and strong women.

We have long needed a new full-length biography of Nightingale. It has been more than 30 years since anyone has risen to the challenge of sifting through newly found letters and stale historiographic debates. And a fabulous one has just appeared in Mark Bostridge's *Florence Nightingale: The Making of an Icon* (2008). Bostridge's Nightingale is neither a heroine nor a harpy. She is a fully formed character who perhaps loved the abstraction of humanity more than the idiosyncrasies of individual humans. Bostridge advances no new thesis or argument about the meaning of Nightingale's life and stunning achievements. Rather, he creates a compelling story of a complicated woman who might well be aghast at how she has come to represent so many different things to so many different people.

Of course, one need not take a particular author's word on any aspect of Nightingale's life. A rich body of work allows Nightingale to speak for herself using her own books and letters to directly engage a reader. Her *Notes on Nursing, Notes on Hospitals,* and *Cassandra* have long been available both as valuable first editions and as more accessible reprints. But her *Suggestions for Thought*, a massive opus privately printed in 1860, never found an audience. The book, her friends told her, needed editing. But it did not find its editors until 1994 when Michael Calabria and Janet Macrae published their *Suggestions for Thought by Florence Nightingale: Selections and Commentaries*. It is one thing to read that Nightingale was well educated, religiously minded, and firmly convinced of the righteousness of her cause. It is quite another to actually experience it and to fully realize the scope of her intellect and the depth of her convictions. I have also particularly enjoyed Martha Vicinus and Bea Nergaard's *Ever Yours, Florence Nightingale: Selected Letters* (1990) and Sue Goldie's *Florence Nightingale: Letters From the Crimea* (1997) for how they document the development of a woman discovering not only how much she loved the taste of official power but also how much good she could do with it.[2] Lynn McDonald's project to publish all of Nightingale's surviving personal letters, professional reports, formal books, and scribbled notes is both more ambitious—and more contentious—than these other collections. Eleven of a projected 16 volumes have been published. McDonald and her collaborators have organized Nightingale's writings thematically rather than chronologically. These volumes allow a reader to trace Nightingale's evolving ideas around such themes as spirituality, the role of women, public health, and Indian reform. But they assume discrete boundaries around particular concerns that may or may not have been apparent to Nightingale, and one does lose a sense of how these selected themes intersected with each other and with the sometimes ordinariness of the life that Nightingale led.[3]

I had once thought that I too might join the pantheon of Nightingale scholars. Fortunately, wise counsel steered me to the then new and exciting work of social historians mining the history of nursing for what it might suggest about the intersections of gender, class, race, work, and the meaning of professionalism in women's lives. Through the 1980s, five scholars, working contemporaneously, defined the field in the United States. Janet Wilson James' "Isabel Hampton and the Professionalization of Nursing in the 1890s" (1979) took a more nuanced look at one of the most important leaders of the American nursing's professionalizing project. Barbara Melosh, by contrast, in *"The Physician's Hand": Work Culture and Conflict in American Nursing* (1982) turned her attention to the heretofore invisible work culture of the vast majority of "ordinary" or "rank and file" nurses and highlighted the power of nurses' craft traditions as they negotiated the often troubled terrain of paid labor. Susan Armeny's 1983 dissertation, *Resolute Enthusiasts: The Effort to Professionalize American Nursing, 1880–1915,* contrasted these women and their concerns about economic security in their day-to-day working lives with the professionalizing ambitions of their ostensible leaders—women like Nutting and Dock—who chose nursing as a way to bring meaning, power, autonomy, and status into their lives. This juxtaposition of craft traditions with professionalizing rhetoric continues to inform some histories of nursing, most recently Tom Olson and Eileen Walsh's *Handling the Sick: The Women of St. Luke's and the Nature of Nursing, 1892–1937* (2004). But Jean Whelan's 2000 dissertation, *Too Many, Too Few: The Supply, Demand, and Distribution of Private Duty Nurses, 1910–1965,* breaks down such divisions and suggests more leadership support for rank-and-file agendas than has been previously acknowledged.

My own work has been more directly framed by Susan Reverby's enormously influential *Ordered to Care: The Dilemma of American Nursing, 1850–1945* (1987). Reverby also positioned nurses as workers. But she framed caring as the most important form of that work and then placed that work within the broader history of the political economy of the evolving American hospital. Her story was one of constraints: of women ordered to care in a society that refused to value caring; and of women caught in the socially constructed bind of perceiving altruism as the antithesis of autonomy and trapped there by class divisions that precluded the development of any new ideology based on gender. Reverby's hard-hitting analysis foregrounded gender and class. Darlene Clark Hine, by contrast, did so with gender and race. Her *Black Women in White: Racial Conflict and Cooperation in the Nursing Profession, 1890–1950* (1989) built on such works as Adah Thoms' *Pathfinders: A History of the Progress of Colored Graduate Nurses* (1985), Mabel Staupers'

No Time for Prejudice; A Story of the Integration of Negroes in Nursing in the United States (1961), and M. Elizabeth Carnegie's multiple editions of *The Path We Tread: Blacks in Nursing Worldwide, 1854–1994* (2000), authors who also figure as important actors in my history. But Hine's study was more conceptual and argued that even as African American nurses contended with their own divisive class issues, they remained joined both by choice and by institutional and social racism to a community beyond that of their hospitals.

Scholars either located across the globe or interested in issues beyond the borders of the United States also experimented with the implications of this "new nursing history." Brian Abel-Smith's *A History of the Nursing Profession* (1975), Christopher Maggs' *The Origins of General Nursing* (1983), Judith Moore's *A Zeal for Responsibility: The Struggle for Professional Nursing in Victorian England, 1868–1883* (1988), and Anne Marie Rafferty's *The Politics of Nursing Knowledge* (1996) brought this perspective to different themes in the history of nursing in the United Kingdom. Katherine McPherson's *Bedside Matters: The Transformation of Canadian Nursing, 1900–1990* (1996) created Canada's first social history of nursing, and Gerard Fealy's *A History of Apprenticeship Nurse Training in Ireland: Bright Faces and Neat Dresses* (2005) did so for Ireland. Joan Lynaugh and Barbara Brush's *Nurses of All Nations: A History of the International Council of Nurses, 1899–1999* (1999) used it to refocus attention on one of the earliest women's international associations.

The role of the state is one emerging theme in these particular histories that begs further analysis. Historians who have studied international communities of nurses with more centralized national governments have long argued that interest in and support for nursing's reform initiatives have often been for reasons that have little to do with only ensuring improvements in health care services. In South Africa, for example, Shula Marks' *Divided Sisterhood: Race, Class and Gender in the South African Nursing Profession* (1994) suggests that the South African state championed the professionalizing aspirations of nursing as a remarkably effective tool to create a stable, bourgeois middle class that might support the policies of the apartheid government. Likewise, Katrin Schultheiss' *Bodies and Souls: Politics and the Professionalization of Nursing in France, 1880–1922* (2001) argues that the government of the Third Republic promoted reforms in nursing education and practice as part of a policy to diminish the influence of the Roman Catholic Church, in general, and the religious nursing sisterhoods, in particular. Catherine Cenzia Choy's *Empire of Care: Nursing and Migration in Filipino American History* (2003) places nurses at the nexus of one country's export economy and another's import one. And Bronwyn Rebekah McFarland-Icke's *Nurses in Nazi Germany: Moral Choice in History* turns caring on its head with nurses as actors in their country's T4 program to extinguish lives not worth living.

But, as studies of nursing in the military show, nurses were never passive victims of state interests. Anne Summers' *Angels and Citizens: British Women as Military Nurses, 1854–1914* (1988) established a new interpretive paradigm in which military nursing corps became the only place where women could participate in the great events of their time in positions of responsibility and personal challenge. This place was not without its own contradictions. Cynthia Toman's *An Officer and a Lady: Canadian Military Nursing and the Second World War* (2007) continues to develop the tensions that existed between commitments to healing within the slaughter of war. Jane Schultz's *Women at the Front: Hospital Workers in Civil War America* (2004) aptly captures the ways groups of women replicated the same race and class hierarchies within the military that they had known in their own communities at home. Mary Sarnecky's encyclopedic *A History of the U.S. Army Nurse Corps* (1999) provides entry into the breath of what were exclusively women's experiences until 1954, when men were also allowed to serve as nurses. Elizabeth Norman's *We Band of Angels: The Untold Story of American Nurses Trapped on Bataan by the Japanese* (1999) and Evelyn Monahan and Rosemary Neidel-Greenlee's *And If I Perish: Frontline U.S. Army Nurses in World War II* (2003) speaks of these women's enduring hold on the public imagination.

The past decade has seen a shift away from interpretive sweeps of time, places, and events to more nuanced analyses of nursing practice. These works seriously engage the constraint and contradiction thesis that has dominated the recent historiography. Yet, they also suggest that such were neither nonnegotiable nor insurmountable. Julie Fairman and Joan Lynaugh's *Critical Care Nursing: A History* (1998) and Julie Fairman's *Making Room in the Clinic: Nurse Practitioners and the Evolution of Modern Health Care* (2008) show how grass-roots alliances with supportive physicians and other health care reformers allowed ambitious nurses to successfully push the boundaries of clinical practice in hospital-based intensive care units and in community-based primary care settings. Margarete Sandelowski's *Devices and Desires: Gender, Technology, and American Nursing* (2000) and Arlene Keeling's *Nursing and the Privilege of Prescription, 1893–2000* (2007) similarly argue that nurses quietly assumed the right to particular practices that physicians believed to be their prerogatives.

Other scholars have turned their attention to areas of nursing work that had long been invisible, and position the practices of their nurses as absolutely central to the larger histories of institutions and of health care practices and policy. Sioban Nelson's *Say Little, Do Much: Nurses, Nuns, and Hospitals in the Nineteenth Century* (2001) and Barbra Mann Wall's *Unlikely Entrepreneurs: Catholic Sisters and the Hospital Marketplace, 1865–1925* (2005) turn to the work of vowed women nurses and give us a more nuanced and gendered story of hospital formation. Joan Lynaugh and Barbara Brush's *American Nursing: From Hospitals to Health Care Systems* (1997) places nurses at the center of the later 20th-century health system movement. Cynthia Connolly, in *Saving Sickly Children: The Tuberculosis Preventorium in American Life, 1909–1970* (2008), places nurses at the nexus of struggles to develop family welfare policies and public health practices for children considered "at risk" of the White Plague of tuberculosis. And Karen Buhler-Wilkerson's *False Dawn: The Rise and Decline of Public Health Nursing, 1900–1930* (1989) and her later *No Place Like Home: A History of Nursing and Home Care in the United States* (2001) draw on the experiences of nurses to examine how the complicated intersections of race, ethnicity, types of illnesses, and the particularities of place influenced who had access to what kinds of care in their own homes. Buhler-Wilkerson's emphasis on place has been particularly influential in my own work.

Biographies have been another important genre. As Laurel Thatcher Ulrich and Emily K. Abel have so brilliantly shown in their respective *A Midwife's Tale: The Life of Martha Ballard, Based on Her Diary, 1785–1812* (1990) and *Hearts of Wisdom: American Women Caring for Kin, 1850–1940* (2000), we now have a richer awareness of the many ways in which women lived their lives enmeshed in the simultaneity of their roles as midwives, nurses, mothers, spouses, neighbors, and friends. We also have a deeper understanding of the ways in which nursing played a very prominent role in the lives of women who are remembered for different kinds of legacies. Elizabeth Pryor's *Clara Barton: Professional Angel* (1988), Ellen Chesler's *Woman of Valor: Margaret Sanger and the Birth Control Movement in America* (1993), and Thomas Brown's *Dorothea Dix: New England Reformer* (1998) all speak to the important place nursing held in these women's lives. Jane Robinson's *Mary Seacole: The Most Famous Black Woman of the Victorian Age* (2004) brings the work of this Jamaican healer out from the glare of Nightingale's lamp. Naomi Rogers' *Healer From the Outback: Sister Elizabeth Kenny, Polio and American Medicine, 1940–1952* (in press) considers the way appropriations of parts of nursing strengthened Kenny's challenge to medical orthodoxy. And, as Nella Larsen's literary reputation has undergone a late 20th-century renaissance, her life and work has been the subject of two biographies: Thadious Davis's *Nella Larsen, Novelist of the Harlem Renaissance: A Woman's Life Unveiled* (1994) and George Hutchinson's *In Search of Nella Larsen: A Biography of the Color Line* (2006). My own interpretation borrows more heavily from Hutchinson, who sharply castigates those like Davis who would demean Larsen's decision to return to nursing when she emerged from seclusion. He, instead, sees it as a sign of strength.

And we can finally look beyond Florence Nightingale if we seek fully developed stories of individual nurses and important work. Judith Godden's *Lucy Osburn, A Lady Displaced: Florence Nightingale's Envoy to Australia* (2006) helps wean us as we make the transition. The best works in this genre use lives lived as nurses to complicate or challenge received wisdom about broader historical themes. Melanie Beals Goan's *Mary Breckinridge: The Frontier Nursing Service & Rural Health in Appalachia* (2008) takes on those who would dismiss the work of Appalachian women reformers as, at best, ineffective and, at worst, destructive, and presents a portrait of achievement within a context of limitations. Similarly, Marjorie Feld's *Lillian Wald: A Biography* (2009) takes issue with the conventional assumption about the American Progressive movement's Anglo-Protestant origins by locating Wald's work in the Jewish ethnic landscape of her time and place. But there are many more stories waiting to be told and ideas to be developed. Possible subjects might be found in anthologies carefully constructed by those keenly aware that nurses have not been well represented in ones about other notable American men and women. Those of note include Martin Kaufman's *Dictionary of American Nursing Biography* (1988) and Vern L. Bullough's three-volume *American Nursing: A Biographical Dictionary* (1988, 1992, 2000).

I join some few others in believing that specifically commissioned histories—most often of associations wishing to document their accomplishments or schools of nursing celebrating particular anniversaries—remain an important and underutilized source. Obviously, my own work acknowledges my debt to alumnae associations who painstakingly created the data I used in my analyses. There are as many of these books as there are states and associations. These books, as a genre, deserve their own analysis for what they might suggest about nursing's sense of self and place. But the best of these individual histories stand as models for how one balances the tensions between data and critical analyses and how one engages audiences bringing different perspectives and expectations to the work. I have particularly enjoyed the ways in which Barbara Brodie has used pictures to tell a story in *Mr. Jefferson's Nurses: The University of Virginia School of Nursing, 1901–2001* (2000) and how Marilyn Flood used documents in her *Promise on Parnassus: The First Century of the UCSF School of Nursing* (2007).

Lamps of the Prairie: A History of Nursing in Kansas (1942/1984), commissioned by the Kansas State Nurses Association and compiled by the Writers'

Program of the Depression-era Works Project Administration, still stands as one of the most important models of this kind of history. It might have languished in relative obscurity, however, had it not been rescued by a reprint series of seminal works in the history of American nursing edited by Susan Reverby and published through the 1980s. In this series, Barbara Melosh introduced readers to an array of evocative short stories about nurses in *American Nurses in Fiction: An Anthology of Short Stories* (1984). Darlene Clark Hine created a compelling collection of documents that had largely been invisible in most accounts of nursing history in *Black Women in the Nursing Profession: A Documentary History* (1985). Reverby herself assembled the reports of an innovative and unusual nursing initiative in *The East Harlem Health Center Demonstration: An Anthology of Pamphlets* (1985). And Karen Buhler-Wilkerson's *Nursing and the Public's Health: An Anthology of Sources* (1989) brought together the seminal articles, surveys, and reports that defined the new field of public health nursing practice. We can look back in time to other anthologies, particularly Annie L. Austin's *A History of Nursing Sourcebook* (1957), a large collection of sources that served as the basis for her own history of nursing. Unfortunately, we cannot yet look ahead to new ones—to ones that will reflect new areas of interest, newly discovered sources, new themes, and the too often invisible actors who have provided most of nursing care.

And for all the histories of schools of nursing, we still know relatively little about the complicated world of nursing education as it worked its way from training schools to universities and from granting diplomas to now conferring doctoral degrees. There are some notable exceptions. Theresa E. Christy's *Cornerstone for Nursing Education, a History of the Division of Nursing Education of Teachers College, Columbia University, 1899–1947* (1969) creates a vivid picture of an institution that played such a pivotal role in the history of nursing, and Patricia Haase's *The Origins and Rise of Associate Degree Nursing Education* (1990) tells of the transformation in nursing education that faculty at Teachers College—albeit unintentionally—helped create in post–World War II America. But the history of education in nursing provides fertile ground for exploring issues in higher education in general. To my mind, it provides a perfect lens through which to consider the ways in which race and class intersected as private and public institutions decided which aspects of nursing education they would support and which they would ignore.

I could go on about what more we need to explore in the history of nursing. We need to know more about the experiences of minorities in nursing. We need to know more about practice and practice politics. But instead I turn to the remarkable resources available to scholars interested in these and other issues in this particular and admittedly small field. The

American Nursing History Archives at Boston University's Gotlieb Archival Research Center holds the official records of the American Nurses Association and the personal papers of many of the formal leaders associated with it. The Barbara Bates Center for the History of Nursing at the University of Pennsylvania, the Center for Nursing Historical Inquiry at the University of Virginia, and the Foundation of the New York State Nurses Association Center for Nursing History boast superb collections of records about more local nursing institutions and organizations. More importantly, they make a concerted effort to be more inclusive in their collecting policies. Their holdings do tell stories of nursing leaders. But they also tell ones of a much more diverse array of individuals with different kinds of contributions to their work and to their communities.

The most exciting sources, I think, have yet to be discovered. Nursing, as I have written, is rooted in and of its communities, and many of the sources I have used are embedded in other kinds of collections scattered throughout the country. Modern technology made my historical research possible. Specialized search engines mining online databases uncovered diaries, letters, and oral histories that would otherwise have passed unnoticed. And I am not even sure that one still needs access to search engines like WorldCat. A simple search for "oral histories of black nurses," for example, yielded a rich array of sources collected by different kinds of groups wanting to document different kinds of experiences. I do not think I will ever see an imagined future where a historian of nursing need not leave home or office to construct a story. However, I do see a future in which technology makes nurses and nursing more visible and encourages more people to bring their own questions about policy and practice to the fascinating world of the care of the sick in their particular communities of interest.

NOTES

1. Dolan began collaborating with Minnie Goodnow on her *History of Nursing* in 1958. Dolan began editing what then became *Goodnow's History of Nursing* in 1960. Dolan subsequently published *Nursing in Society: A Historical Perspective* in 1968 and took it through 13 editions until she herself turned to M. Louise Fitzpatrick and Eleanor Kron Herrmann as collaborators in 1983. Saunders (Philadelphia) published all these editions.
2. Parts of this evaluation come from reviews I have written of these books.
3. A description of the project and the volumes are available through Wilfrid Laurier University Press. Retrieved from http://www.sociology.uoguelph.ca/fnightingale/

REFERENCES

Abel-Smith, B. (1975). *A history of the nursing profession*. London: Heinemann.
Armeny, S. (1983). *Resolute enthusiasts: The effort to professionalize American nursing, 1880–1915*. Columbia, MO: University of Missouri.
Ashley, J. A. (1976). *Hospitals, paternalism and the role of the nurse*. New York, NY: Teachers College Press.
Austin, A. L. (1957). *A history of nursing sourcebook*. New York, NY: Putnam.
Baly, M. (1997). *Florence Nightingale and the nursing legacy*. London, UK: Whurr Publishers.
Bostridge, M. (2008). *Florence Nightingale: The making of an icon*. New York, NY: Farrar, Straus and Giroux.
Brodie, B. (2000). *Mr. Jefferson's nurses: The University of Virginia School of Nursing, 1901–2001*. Charlottesville, VA: University of Virginia Press.
Brown, T. (1998). *Dorothea Dix: New England reformer*. Cambridge, MA: Harvard University Press.
Buhler-Wilkerson, K. (1989). *Nursing and the public's health: An anthology of sources*. New York, NY: Garland Press.
Bullough, V. L. (1988). *American nursing: A biographical dictionary* (Vol. I). New York, NY: Garland Publishing.
Bullough, V. L. (1992). *American nursing: A biographical dictionary* (Vol. II). New York, NY: Garland Publishing.
Bullough, V. L. (2000). *American nursing: A biographical dictionary* (Vol. III). New York, NY: Springer Publishing.
Bullough, V., Bullough, B., & Stanton, M. (Eds.). (1990). *Florence Nightingale and her era: A collection of new scholarship*. New York, NY: Garland Press.
Calabria, M., & Macrae, J. (1994). *Suggestions for thought by Florence Nightingale: Selections and commentaries*. Philadelphia, PA: University of Pennsylvania Press.
Carnegie, M. E. (2000). *The path we tread: Blacks in nursing worldwide* (3rd ed.). Sudbury, MA: Jones and Bartlett.
Chesler, E. (1993). *Woman of valor: Margaret Sanger and the birth control movement in America*. New York, NY: Anchor Books.
Choy, C. C. (2003). *Empire of care: Nursing and migration in Flipino American history*. Durham, NC: Duke University Press.
Connolly, C. (2008). *Saving sickly children: The tuberculosis preventorium in American life, 1909–1970*. New Brunswick, NJ: Rutgers University Press.
Davis, T. M. (1994). *Nella Larsen, novelist of the Harlem renaissance: A woman's life unveiled*. Baton Rouge, LA: Louisiana State University Press.
Dock, L., & Stewart, I. (1920). *A short history of nursing*. New York, NY: G. P. Putnam's Sons.
Fairman, J. (2008). *Making room in the clinic: Nurse practitioners and the evolution of modern health care*. New Brunswick, NJ: Rutgers University Press.
Fairman, J., & Lynaugh, J. E. (1998). *Critical care nursing: A history*. Philadelphia, PA: University of Pennsylvania Press

Fealy, G. (2005). *A history of apprenticeship nurse training in Ireland: Bright faces and neat dresses*. London: Routledge.

Feld, M. (2009). *Lillian Wald: A biography*. Chapel Hill, NC: University of North Carolina Press.

Flood, M. (2007). *Promise on Parnassus: The first century of the UCSF School of Nursing*. San Francisco, CA: University of California San Francisco Press.

Gill, G. (2004). *Nightingales: The extraordinary upbringing and curious life of Miss Florence Nightingale*. New York, NY: Ballantine Books.

Goan, M. B. (2008). *Mary Breckinridge: The frontier nursing service & rural health in Appalachia*. Chapel Hill, NC: University of North Carolina Press.

Godden, J. (2006). *Lucy Osburn, a lady displaced: Florence Nightingale's envoy to Australia*. Sydney, AU: Sydney University Press.

Goldie, S. (1997). *Florence Nightingale: Letters from the Crimea*. Manchester, UK: University of Manchester Press.

Gourlay, J. (2003). *Florence Nightingale and the health of the Raj*. Surrey, UK: Ashgate.

Hamilton, D. (1994). Constructing the mind of nursing. *Nursing History Review*, 2, 3–28.

Hine, D. C. (1989). *Black women in white: Racial conflict and cooperation in the nursing profession, 1890–1950*. New York, NY: Macmillan.

Hutchinson, G. (2006). *In search of Nella Larsen: A biography of the color line*. Cambridge, MA: Harvard University Press.

James, J. W. (1979). Isabel Hampton and the professionalization of nursing in the 1890s. In M. J. Vogel & C. E. Rosenberg (Eds.), *The Therapeutic Revolution* (pp. 201–244). Philadelphia, PA: University of Pennsylvania Press.

Kalish, P. A., & Kalish, B. J. (1986). *The advance of American nursing* (3rd ed.). Philadelphia, PA: J.B. Lippincott.

Kansas State Nurses Association. (1942/1984). *Lamps of the prairie: A history of nursing in Kansas*. New York, NY: Garland reprint, Garland Publishing.

Kaufman, M. (1988). *Dictionary of American nursing biography*. New York, NY: Garland Publishing.

Keeling, A. (2007). *Nursing and the privilege of prescription, 1893–2000*. Columbus, OH: The Ohio State University Press.

Lynaugh, J., & Brush, B. (1997). *American nursing: From hospitals to health care systems*. Hoboken, NJ: Wiley-Blackwell.

Lynaugh, J., & Brush, B. (Eds.). (1999). *Nurses of all nations: A history of the international council of nurses, 1899–1999*. Philadelphia, PA: Williams and Wilkins Publishers.

Maggs, C. (1983). *The origins of general nursing*. London, UK: Croom Helm.

Marks, S. (1994). *Divided sisterhood: Race, class and gender in the South African nursing profession*. London, UK: Palgrave Macmillan.

McFarland-Icke, B. R. (1999). *Nurses in Nazi Germany: Moral choice in history*. Princeton, NJ: Princeton University Press.

McPherson, K. (1996). *Bedside matters: The transformation of Canadian nursing, 1900–1990*. Toronto: Oxford University Press.

Melosh, B. (1982). *"The physician's hand": Work culture and conflict in American nursing*. Philadelphia, PA: Temple University Press.

Melosh, B. (1984). *American nurses in fiction: An anthology of short stories.* New York, NY: Garland Publishing.

Monahan, E. M., & Neidel-Greenlee, R. (2003). *And if I perish: Frontline U.S. army nurses in World War II.* New York, NY: Knopf.

Moore, J. (1988). *A zeal for responsibility: The struggle for professional nursing in Victorian England, 1868–1883.* Athens, GA: University of Georgia Press.

Nelson, S. (2001). *Say little, do much: Nurses, nuns, and hospitals in the nineteenth century.* Philadelphia, PA: University of Pennsylvania Press.

Norman, E. (1999). *We band of angels: The untold story of American nurses trapped on Bataan by the Japanese.* New York, NY: Random House.

Nutting, M. A., & Dock, L. L. (1907). *A history of nursing* (Vol. I). New York, NY: G. P. Putnam's Sons.

Olson, T., & Walsh, E. (2004). *Handling the sick: The women of St. Luke's and the nature of nursing, 1892–1937.* Columbus, OH: The Ohio State University Press.

Poovey, M. (1988). *Uneven developments: The ideological work of gender in Mid-Victorian England* (pp. 13–15). Chicago, IL: University of Chicago Press.

Pryor, E. (1988). *Clara Barton: Professional angel.* Philadelphia, PA: University of Pennsylvania Press.

Rafferty, A. M. (1996). *The politics of nursing knowledge.* London, UK: Routledge.

Reverby, S. (1985). *The East Harlem health center demonstration: An anthology of pamphlets.* New York, NY: Garland Publishing.

Reverby, S. M. (1987). *Ordered to care: The dilemma of American nursing, 1850–1945.* New York, NY: Cambridge University Press.

Robinson, J. (2004). *Mary Seacole: The most famous Black woman of the Victorian age.* New York, NY: Carroll & Graf.

Rogers, N. (In press). *Healer from the outback: Sister Elizabeth Kenny, polio and American medicine, 1940–1952.* New York, NY: Oxford University Press.

Sandelowski, M. (2000). *Devices and desires: Gender, technology, and American nursing.* Chapel Hill, NC: University of North Carolina Press.

Sarnecky, M. T. (1999). *A history of the U.S. Army Nurse Corps.* Philadelphia, PA. University of Pennsylvania Press.

Schultheiss, K. (2001). *Bodies and souls: Politics and the professionalization of nursing in France, 1880–1922.* Cambridge, MA: Harvard University Press.

Schultz, J. E. (2004). *Women at the front: Hospital workers in Civil War America.* Chapel Hill, NC: University of North Carolina Press.

Small, H. (1999). *Florence Nightingale: Avenging angel.* New York, NY: St. Martin's Press.

Smith, F. B. (1982). *Florence Nightingale: Reputation and power.* London, UK: Croom Helm.

Staupers, M. K. (1961). *No time for prejudice: A story of the integration of Negroes in nursing in the United States.* New York, NY: Macmillan.

Summers, A. (1988). *Angels and citizens: British women as military nurses, 1854–1914.* London, UK: Routledge & Kegan Paul.

Swenson, K. (2005). *Medical women and Victorian fiction.* Columbia, MI: The University of Missouri Press.

Thoms, A. (1985). *Pathfinders: A history of the progress of colored graduate students.* New York, NY: Garland Publishing.

Toman, C. (2007). *An officer and a lady: Canadian military nursing and the Second World War.* Vancouver, CA: University of British Columbia Press.

Vicinus, M., & Nergaard, B. (Eds.). (1990). *Ever yours, Florence Nightingale: Selected letters.* Cambridge, MA: Harvard University Press.

Wall, B. M. (2005). *Unlikely entrepreneurs: Catholic sisters and the hospital marketplace, 1865–1925.* Columbus, OH: Ohio State University Press.

Whelan, J. C. (2000). *Too many, too few: The supply, demand, and distribution of private duty nurses, 1910–1965* (PhD dissertation). University of Pennsylvania, Philadelphia, PA: University of Pennsylvania.

Wilkerson, B. (2001). *False dawn and no place like home: A history of nursing and home care in the United States.* Baltimore, MD: The Johns Hopkins University Press.

Woodham-Smith, C. (1950). *Florence Nightingale, 1820–1910.* London, UK: Constable Press.

COMMENTARY: INTERVIEW WITH DR. BARBRA MANN WALL

Mary de Chesnay

The study of history gives us a framework for understanding our present and future. Those nurses who study history give the rest of us a fascinating framework for understanding the rich traditions and influences on our profession. In the preceding chapter, Dr. D'Antonio provides us with many references that describe the state of the art of literature by those who document nursing history. I wish I had read Dr. D'Antonio's work as a graduate student because she inspires us to look at our past in a different light. For example, while reading about the history of nursing to prepare this volume, I discovered to my surprise that both Harriet Tubman and Louisa May Alcott were nurses in the American Civil War. Tubman is best known for her work in the Underground Railroad, but less so for her nursing the former slaves-turned-Union soldiers. A contemporary of Tubman wrote that she had been recruited and appointed by the surgeon general of the time (Bradford, 1886). In her memoirs, Alcott describes her journey to the war, her challenges as a woman traveling alone and trying to obtain her documents, and her perceptions of caring for the wounded (Alcott, 1863).

This volume provides other kinds of historical research examples that show the breadth of scholarship of nurse historians. One such scholar is Dr. Barbra Mann Wall, a nurse who obtained her doctorate in history and wrote about the tradition of Catholic hospitals and their role in the development of the profession. In an attempt to grasp the essence of historical research, I interviewed Dr. Wall, who commented briefly on current trends and sources and offered advice to those who wish to conduct historical research.

MdC: What do you think is the current trend, focus, or importance of historical research conducted by nurses—that is, what makes it so exciting right now?

BW: Race, class, and gender have always been issues. African Americans were not allowed in the American Nurses Association until 1950. Current students don't know our history. In medicine it was different. The doctors were united, but nurses fight each other. Examples are the different degrees we have: diploma, associate degree, baccalaureate degree. As an alternative, Fairman's work showed how nurse practitioners aligned themselves with physicians. My study of Catholic traditions showed nursing long before Florence Nightingale. But I would say history can help us understand health policy. Look at how nurses contextualize nursing and health.

MdC: What are the one or two sources novices (that is, nursing PhD students) should read as an example of historical research (e.g., certainly *Nursing History Review* articles)?

BW: I would recommend Connelly's study of TB sanatoriums. *Ordered to Care* is a classic. Lavinia Dock looked at tensions in nursing. Julie's [Fairman] book on critical care, mine on American Catholic hospitals. I looked at gender issues. And Pat D'Antonio's *American Nursing* (2010).

MdC: What advice would you give nurses who want to conduct historical research?

BW: Some nurses obtain a PhD in history like I did, others hold degrees in nursing but have taken history courses in the PhD programs (e.g., Penn [University of Pennsylvania]—they focus on history, but others attend schools that don't have history [graduate courses]). I suggest they take courses in their local history departments. Some funding sources are the American Nurses' Foundation, Sigma Theta Tau, and the National Library of Medicine. The main advice is that history is fun! Each chapter tells a story.

REFERENCES

Alcott, L. M. (1863). *Hosptial sketches*. Boston, MA: James Redpath, Publisher.
Bradford, S. (1886). *Harriet: The Moses of her people*. New York, NY: Geo/R. Lockwood & Son.
Connolly, C. A. (2008). *Saving sickly children: The tuberculosis preventorium in American life, 1909–1970*. New Brunswick, NJ: Rutgers University Press.
D'Antonio, P. (2010). *American nursing: A history of knowledge, authority and the meaning of work*. Baltimore, MD: Johns Hopkins University Press.
Dock, L., & Stewart, I. (1920). *A short history of nursing*. New York, NY: G.P. Putnam's Sons.
Fairman, J. (2008) *Making room in the clinic: Nurse practitioners and the evolution of modern health care*. New Brunswick, NJ: Rutgers Press.
Reverby, S. (1987). *Ordered to care: The dilemma of American nursing, 1850–1945 (Cambridge Studies in the History of Medicine)*. Cambridge, UK: Cambridge University Press.
Wall, B. M. (2005). *Unlikely entrepreneurs: Catholic sisters and the hospital marketplace, 1865–1925*. Columbus, OH: Ohio State University Press.

Chapter Three

Inside Track of Doing Historical Research: My Dissertation Story

Annemarie McAllister and Sandra B. Lewenson

> *Pioneering requires imagination and foresight.*
> —McManus to Arnold, January 9, 1953, p. 3

The rich and storied history of the Division of Nursing Education at Teachers College (TC), Columbia University, is a testament to the strength of the nurse leaders at its helm. Dr. R. Louise McManus became the first non-Canadian director of the division in 1947, following in the footsteps of M. Adelaide Nutting and Isabel Maitland Stewart. As one of the few nurses in the country at the time to have a doctorate, McManus was at the helm of TC's Division of Nursing Education for 14 years before retiring in 1961. Under her leadership, remarkable progress was made in the world of nursing education (Champagne, 1981).

It was this remarkable progress in the world of nursing education that piqued my (Annemarie McAllister's) interest in the development of the associate degree model for the education of nurses, its two architects (R. Louise McManus and Mildred Montag), and the influence of the TC milieu, which resulted in the completion of my dissertation utilizing the historical methodology (McAllister, 2012). This chapter tells my story as I developed an interest in the history of nursing and began to formulate questions for doctoral studies that could only be answered by using historical analysis. I write this chapter from a personal perspective and therefore write in the first person to convey this experience. The chapter walks us through the various stages or steps that led me to successfully complete my dissertation examining the education of nurses using the historical method (McAllister, 2012). This chapter follows many of the headings from Chapter 1 in this monograph so that the reader, interested in doing historical research, can learn from my experience. I include my experiences with choosing a topic, developing questions, assessing available resources, learning the method, attending conferences, meeting and networking with historians, writing for institutional review board (IRB) and grants, visiting archives, analyzing the data, writing the narrative, meeting with advisors, and figuring out when to stop. Also in this chapter, the relationship between the advisors selected to support the development of the dissertation will emerge as well because this was relevant to finishing on time and accomplishing my goal. If history is perceived as a story, I begin with my story as it began long before my doctoral work at TC, and plays a strong role in my choice of topic, method, and analysis.

IN THE BEGINNING

My nursing education began at Bronx Community College (BCC) in the Bronx, a borough of New York City. This school began its associate degree program in nursing in the early 1960s as an outcome of the work of Mildred Montag, a TC faculty member and architect of the associate degree model. I attended BCC from 1975 to 1977 directly out of high school. With no guidance from my guidance counselor, my plan was to complete school as soon as possible so I could get a job and get my own apartment. This is indeed what happened. The 2-year degree enabled me to enter into my adult life quicker than I would have had I gone through a 4-year program. At that time, 2-year associate degree programs were in the second decade of their existence and quite popular with guidance counselors (at my school at least), who encouraged young women to enter nursing training via this route. Despite this, I was strongly encouraged by BCC College faculty to continue on into a baccalaureate program because it was believed that, by 1985, the baccalaureate degree would be the minimum requirement (American Nurses' Association, 1965). The faculty was responding to nursing's effort to move nursing education away from the technical model and the diploma model towards a baccalaureate education for all nurses. And I believed them. It is important to note here that at the time City University of New York (CUNY) was tuition free for all residents of New York City, and was free up until my second year at BCC in 1976. Nevertheless, the cost was minimal in comparison to private institutions in the area. My education was affordable because I continued to work through college with the same job I held while in high school.

As the faculty suggested, I immediately enrolled at the 4-year Herbert H. Lehman College in the Bronx, another part of the CUNY system, which awarded a bachelor of science degree in nursing. The program I attended was geared for people like me who had completed an associate degree in nursing. We were all practicing nurses, we had sat for the licensure exam (then called state boards), and we were all working in clinical settings. I worked as a staff nurse in the emergency room at Montefiore Hospital, a large urban medical center in the Bronx. By day, I was a student sitting with other students—the younger generic class and the RNs returning like me. By evening I was back on staff working as a nurse. Lehman kept challenging the RN students and their nursing skills and former coursework. They required us to repeat nursing courses, such as nutrition and growth and development, which we had already taken in our associate degree programs. In reflective hindsight, the faculty was just trying to give us what it felt was missing from the associate degree curriculum. At the time, however, I was becoming disillusioned, but was able to successfully complete the courses that they wanted me to repeat. I attended as a part-time student and finished my degree in 1983, just under the supposed 1985 deadline when all nurses were to have been required to have the bachelor's degree to enter the field (American Nurses' Association, 1965).

It took me 23 more years to consider returning to school for a master's degree. The doctorate had not yet entered my mind. I was working in a cardiac setting at Columbia University in New York City while raising a family and getting older. My work setting offered a tuition benefit that I could not ignore, and subsequently I applied for and was accepted into the Executive Program for Nurses, a master's program at TC, Columbia University, from which I graduated in 2008. Not wanting to stop, I continued on in the school and entered the doctoral cohort group beginning that same year. Thus began my quest for a dissertation topic and the start of my journey down the road to becoming a nurse historian.

Developing an Interest in History

The journey for the doctoral student not only includes the coursework but also the constant worry about choosing a dissertation topic. "Choose a topic you like," I was told. "Choose something that you can get done in a reasonable time frame," another said. "Think of it as a really big paper," another offered. My research experience and subsequent publications included only quantitative research with a very narrow focus and a collection of numerical data that hopefully yielded an unbiased result that could somehow be generalized to other populations. I assumed that my dissertation topic would be quantitative. This was my research experience—my history, one would say. Like most nurses, I was comfortable with the clarity and organization that a quantitative approach required, but yet I was interested in the depth and breadth that history offered, and I was ready to make a change.

Several things led me to develop an interest in the history of nursing, specifically, an interest in TC and its influence over the mid-20th century nursing education and practice. It began when one of my professors, Dr. Sheila Melli, spoke to the doctoral cohort and emphatically said, "There is such a richness of nursing here at *Teachers College*." As there is a dearth of courses in nursing history in most nursing school curricula, my interest was piqued. I had been in the master's cohort at TC and heard Melli previously speak about this rich history, including some of the nursing giants who had attended college here and then were faculty, like Hildegard Peplau, Virginia Henderson, Martha Rogers, and others. Peplau's name rang a bell for me, most likely from my psychiatric rotation, when I was a nursing student at BCC in the Bronx. I quickly found her biography and intended to read the portion related to her years at TC, but found myself immersed in her story (Callaway, 2002). Melli's comment stayed with me as I moved into the doctoral cohort, where we met every Friday for a full day of classes and constantly worried about choosing a dissertation topic and completing the work within some kind of reasonable timeframe.

Value of Historical Research

My discovery that a TC doctoral student, Mildred Montag, completed her dissertation by suggesting the associate degree model (Montag, 1950) led to my dissertation topic. Finally I was on my way. Montag's original research resulted in the sudden explosion of associate degree programs in community and junior colleges throughout the United States. Because I was an associate degree graduate, I had a keen interest in how this happened. What I really wanted to know was how did Montag get this done so fast in a profession that seems to proceed at a snail's pace. I wanted to know more about Montag: who she worked with, who influenced her, and how they managed to successfully put forth the associate degree model in a scant 9 years. Melli's words about the richness of history at TC resounded as I started this exploration.

Mildred Montag was a doctoral student at TC under the tutelage of R. Louise McManus, then the director of the department of nursing education. McManus was Montag's dissertation advisor and was in the habit of keeping ideas for research projects in what was known as the "bottom drawer" of her desk (Schorr & Zimmerman, 1988). When she found someone she considered a worthy student, a project appeared, often with funding provided.

In this particular case, Montag had an interest in curriculum development, and McManus had a project in mind. The project entailed developing a curriculum for a 2-year nursing degree that would take place in the nation's community colleges, then called junior colleges. During the post–World War II period, the looming shortage of qualified nurses was apparent in the same time frame when the nation was moving away from an agrarian society to a more technologically oriented populace. The Truman Commission examined the status of education in the United States and proposed a 2-year post–high school education for the majority of Americans (President's Commission on Higher Education, 1946).

Nursing educators were consistently interested in moving the education of nurses into the nation's collegiate system, and the concomitant growth of the nations' junior colleges excited interest in some of the faculty at TC. The role of TC, arguably considered the premier school of graduate education for nurses, cannot be understated in the propulsion of Montag's (1950) dissertation topic titled, *Education of Nursing Technicians. A Report of a Type B Project*. Her dissertation was published almost verbatim in 1951 and outlined a curriculum for a 2-year program in nursing education. She used the term *technicians*, which met with resistance from others in nursing. At this time, McManus was questioned by philanthropist Mary Rockefeller about what TC was doing about the nursing shortage. McManus responded by opening that bottom drawer and presenting a faster and possibly more economical route into the practice of nursing. This was the same proposal that was the basis of Montag's dissertation and led to funding to the extent of $23,000 to experiment with the cooperative research project. This was an experiment that caught on and changed the face of nursing education, whereby community colleges clamored for this opportunity to start nursing programs on their campuses. Montag (1959) published the result of this larger experiment, which found that students educated in these programs performed as well as, or better than, traditionally diploma educated and even baccalaureate educated nurses. By the time the results were published in 1959, there were more nursing programs in community colleges outside of the original eight sites mentioned in the research project than there were inside. It can be said that this model was one of the first and, perhaps, the only educational model that was based on research. The associate degree model of nursing education was off and running in a matter of 9 years. The effort to stem the shortage of nurses, along with the desire of nurse leaders to move the education of nurses into the collegiate system of higher education, became a reality, but not without controversy and unintended consequences that still stymie the profession today. The cry to require the baccalaureate degree as the minimum requirement for entry into the practice of nursing first sounded in 1965 and went unheeded, as the associate degree remains the primary avenue into the profession. Montag and McManus's success in putting forth the associate degree model dwarfed the growth of baccalaureate programs in the United States and has become one of the most contentious issues that the profession still grapples with today, more than 60 years later.

The desire to examine and preserve the history of issues and events in the development of the education of nurses resulted from my curiosity about what made nurse leaders such as McManus, Montag, and others do what they did. The story of how that occurred is long, and my research is but a small portion of that story. Using a historical methodology serves to connect today's past with tomorrow's future. It is a small part of the story, but one that enables us to see how the progression in nursing education evolved and provides insight into future possibilities as the nursing profession continues to struggle with the entry into practice issue (McAllister, 2012).

Evolution of My Becoming a Nurse Historian

The Importance of Collegial Networking

One of my colleagues in the cohort asked, "Did you know that there is a website that lists the gravesites of famous nurses?" That sounded both bizarre and interesting to me and led me to the discovery of the American Association for the History of Nursing (AAHN), an organization that I would soon become well acquainted with, and on whose board I would subsequently (several years later, now) serve. Initially, I had been doing research on nurse-to-nurse hostility; however, my colleagues in the doctoral cohort said that that was "too mean." I had done a great deal of work on this topic and the quantitative method, but it was not where I wanted to go in my doctoral studies. We spoke about our educational trajectory in nursing—mine being in the associate program followed by the RN-BS program at Lehman College. I had never looked at the RN-BS program like a groundbreaking program at the time, until my colleague at TC said to me: "You went to an RN-BS program in the late 1970s? That must have been groundbreaking back then." I was a full-time working nurse when I went back to this RN-BSN program, and I did not consider it to be groundbreaking or of any historical significance. I knew I was different than the generic students who had time to spend in the cafeteria, time to walk around the campus, and time to be a student. I was an adult learner who went back for a baccalaureate.

That same colleague handed me a book, *Cornerstone for Nursing Education* by Teresa Christy (1969), which outlined the first 50 years of the department of nursing education at TC. "Here read this," she said. "It's a real page turner." I did and she was right. That's when I thought, "Ohh… I should write about the next 50 years starting with R. Louise McManus, Montag's advisor and the director of the program!" The combination of reading Christy's book and learning how McManus was Montag's mentor led me to consider my next move to study the history of the McManus years at TC.

Exposure to Nurse Historians

The exposure to other nurse historians is an important part of the journey of doing historical research. During this time period, the famous nurse historian Sandy Lewenson came as a guest lecturer to TC, and this was fortuitous for me. Her class on historical methodology was informative and immensely interesting for me. Her presentation included historical photographs, all of which I found raised more questions about the people who preceded me at TC and in nursing. It wasn't necessarily her topic that convinced me to use the historical method, but rather the "oldness" of the photos, the stories, and the connections with topics today. She spoke about nurse leaders that my colleagues and I were not familiar with but certainly added to the richness and color that Melli spoke about earlier. After this class, the director of the doctoral program, Elaine LaMonica Riglosa, suggested that I contact Lewenson to discuss doing a historical study. When she said this, I said to myself, "Why would she want to help me?" That's when my colleague in the cohort kindly explained to me the value of including the statement, "TC doctoral student" in the subject lines of my exploratory e-mails. I used this line to contact Sandy Lewenson, whom I subsequently asked to be my chair, and the noted historian Louise Fitzpatrick, Dean of the Villanova School of Nursing, who shared her memories as a student and faculty member at TC in a subsequent oral history.

Melli, who at this point was an important mentor to me, also recommended that I meet the Chief Program Officer of the National League for Nurses (then president of the NLN) Elaine Tagliareni, as well as community college educator Elizabeth Speakman, both former Melli students who had completed a historical video on Mildred Montag (Tagliareni & Speakman, 1999). Melli, Talgiareni, and I met for lunch to discuss possible dissertation topics, as I was interested in the associate degree and Montag's involvement. Each of the historians that I met provided me with additional contacts, which were helpful to me as I began my research in earnest.

Importance of Networking With Historians

Lewenson advised me to join the AAHN. With that membership, she also encouraged me to attend the fall annual meeting; that year it was to be held in Egham, UK. Boschma (2009) notes the importance of attending conferences and sharing and networking with other historians. The AAHN international conference included a luncheon for doctoral students. At the international meeting, the noted historian Cynthia Connolly led the group, and at a later conference, Arlene Keeling, Dean at the University of Virginia School of Nursing, shared her insights on the dissertation process. These meetings were invaluable. It was at these luncheons, held as roundtable discussions, where students discussed their historical research and where they were in the process. It was helpful to hear what others were doing, how they found their resources, how they felt while doing the research, where they found their support, and to hear their suggestions for my own research.

It was not just the formal presentations and luncheons that provided rich support for my research. It was through meeting historians and other doctoral students—informally in the cafeteria, the conference hallways, and on the bus to events, where we shared our stories and our research, both our successes and our foibles—that I found a willingness among these seasoned nurse historians to share their expertise and their contact information if I had questions. One historian led me to another, and I met all the "greats" of the period, as well as people whose books I had read, and those whose books were waiting to be read. Joy Buck, for example, was one of the first historians I was introduced to, and she acknowledged my interest in studying nursing history. Gertje Boschma and Sonya Grympa, two noted oral historians, both had long discussions with me about my research. There was no better introduction to doing historical research than what these conversations provided. I was welcomed into this group and felt I belonged.

LEARNING THE METHOD

Deciding to research a historical topic for my doctoral dissertation required me to start from scratch. The first step was to learn about the historical method, a method that is decidedly nonlinear and fraught with uncertainty. Lewenson and Herrmann (2008) outlined the skills necessary to do historical research in *Capturing Nursing History: A Guide to Historical Methods in Research*. This text was helpful as I attempted to stay organized. The AAHN website includes a bibliography of other references on the historical method.

Questions were raised: Are there enough resources for the topic I want to study? Is this a worthwhile topic? Does anyone know about this topic? Has someone done this research before? These are the questions that plagued me in my uncertainty. I addressed these questions by beginning my library and Internet search; this brought me to the archives of TC, which are found only online.

The Importance of Archives

The exploration of archives is key to the development of the historian's research both in assessing the availability of primary and secondary sources and the costs and time associated with traveling to these facilities. Many archives have finding aids that can be accessed online. This helps the student determine if the available materials are appropriate for the study in question. My own research started with the Nutting Collection at TC, Columbia University, Gottesman Library (www.library.tc.columbia.edu). This is an extensive digitized collection of materials related to the department of nursing education at TC and contains materials related to the development of nursing education.

In addition to the TC archives, other related materials were located at the University of Pennsylvania Barbara Bates Center for Study of the History of Nursing (www.nursing.upenn.edu/history/Pages/default.aspx); the Rockefeller Archives in Pocantico, New York (www.rockarch.org); and the Adelphi University Library (www.libraries.adelphi.edu/archives-and-special-collections/contact-us). The archives of interest were found by suggestions from my dissertation committee, simple Google searches, and from references gleaned from scholarly articles and previous historical dissertations. In fact, one of the first steps I took when I was considering a historical topic was to locate and read historical dissertations in my own institution. This was helpful in two ways: first, to see what it took to complete an entire project, and second, to assess my interest in completing a dissertation using the historical method. TC has a long history of doctoral candidates with an interest in the history of nursing; although not all graduate programs share such a propensity for historical research, I would recommend this step for any student trying to decide on a dissertation topic no matter which graduate program he or she attends. My reading led me to other resources that were helpful to me when I was trying to narrow down my topic.

Each archive has its own rules and requirements. Many have finding aids online that allow the researcher to assess the availability of materials related to his or her topic as well as materials from the same time frame that can help add context to the research. For example, many of the materials I accessed at the Rockefeller archive were related not only to my topic of the education of nurses but also to funding initiatives that the Rockefeller foundation prioritized in the mid-20th century, which were related to the health of the American populace. The archive required a detailed explanation of the researcher's proposed study to be submitted in writing to an archivist at the facility. The archivist would then assess the availability of materials and also suggest related items before setting up an appointment to visit the archive. The Rockefeller facility is a world-renowned organization that is visited by scholars from around the world. Summertime was particularly busy as many academics scheduled their research time during the summer months. Scheduling visits required time off from work and estimating how much time an individual needed to assess the materials. Once I obtained research time at the archive, I was given a tour of the facility, a stunning mansion built by John D. Rockefeller for his wife Mary, who never actually lived there. Each researcher is assigned his or her own desk and a cart is brought in containing the requested materials. The rules are explained, as many of the materials are originals and fragile; thus, they require careful handling. As a novice historian, this was an enlightening experience, and the major difficulty became trying to stay on task and not read everything!

One of the timesavers was the use of a digital camera or cell phone to take pictures of materials that were of interest for later reading. The volume of some of the papers was simply too long to read at one sitting. Of the utmost importance was the documentation of the source materials; the archivist provided slips of paper to fill out for each item that could then be placed under the edge of the material to be photographed, thus remaining visible for future citation information. There is nothing more disconcerting than coming down the home stretch of completing your dissertation and finding that you cannot use some material because of a lack of proper citation. Revisiting the archive to find the reference can be really time consuming.

When I was at Rockefeller Archives, I ran into noted historian Patricia D'Antonio, who, coincidentally, was there doing research for some of her work. She immediately asked me about my research topic and was very encouraging. Receiving this kind of encouragement was wonderful for a beginning researcher like me, and served as an example of the role that seasoned historians play in developing new nurse historians.

My experience at the Adelphi Archive was different and exciting in other ways. My query to the librarian resulted in an enthusiastic response from an archivist who was not only familiar with my topic but also had had contact with Mildred Montag.

The Adelphi School of Nursing was started in the late 1940s with the recruitment of Mildred Montag, then a doctoral student at TC, who became the first director of the program; incidentally, this was the first program for nursing on Long Island, New York (Safier, 1977). The collection of papers and photos from this era were contained in the basement of one of the dormitories and the archivist was happy to have me examine them and give me a tour of the campus.

On January 1, 1943, Mildred Montag became the first director of the School of Nursing at Adelphi College. It was wartime, and there was a shortage of nurses. In that first year, approximately 25 students were admitted as part of the Nurse Training Act of 1943, also called the Bolton Act, which provided federal funding of more than $45 million to establish the United States Cadet Nurse Corps. By the time Montag left Adelphi 5 years later to continue her doctoral studies at TC, the program had graduated more than 500 students ("65 Years of Caring," 2009).

The program grew quickly as a result of the Bolton Act, and the college, for the first time, found itself in need of dormitories. Adelphi was a commuter college at the time, but the desire to recruit nursing students from a wide geographical area and the availability of government construction grants spurred dormitory construction. The opening of the two dormitories for women in 1944 was celebrated with much pomp and circumstance. Many dignitaries attended the event, and the First Lady of the United States, Eleanor Roosevelt, delivered an address to the crowd entitled, "The Challenge of Nursing for Young Women Today" ("65 Years of Caring," 2009). In her address to the Cadet Corps on the occasion of the dedication of the two new buildings, Mrs. Roosevelt congratulated them on their choice to help the country in a time of war both abroad near battle sites and at home, helping returning soldiers face what she called their second fight.

The archivist took me on a tour of those two buildings as well as the Mildred Montag memorial garden that was in a prominent position outside the student life building on this beautiful campus. The sight of the dormitories brought to life the scene in the photos of the dedication ceremony, which I had access to in the archive.

My query to the Barbara Bates Center for the Study of the History of Nursing at the University of Pennsylvania was enthusiastically received. The response I received indicated that my research question was circulated among the faculty there for input and suggestions. I attended one of the Bates Center Seminars and met some of the wonderful, well-published historians on the faculty like Joan Lynaugh, Julie Fairman, Jean Whelan, Cindy Connolly, Barbra Mann Wall, and Pat D'Antonio. These people are well known in the world of nursing history, and yes, there is a world of nursing history. The Bates Center is one of the centers of that world. The opportunity to receive input from noted nurse historians was invaluable.

Another noted center, devoted to supporting historical scholarship in nursing, is located at the University of Virginia, where noted nurse historian Arlene Keeling is the director. Recently renamed the Eleanor Crowder Bjoring Center for Nursing Historical Inquiry, this archive is a great place to do research and meet historians on faculty like Keeling, Mary Gibson, and Professor Emerita Barbara Brodie. Although I did not use this center for my dissertation, it's on my radar for future studies. The area itself is historical and steeped in the history of our country.

There are many other archival collections available for researchers interested in the history of nursing. The previous examples constitute the tip of the iceberg. Simple Google searches can help locate resources. Many will send copies of materials for a fee. This can help control the costs associated with travel to distant sites. Also, again, check out the AAHN website for a full list of archival collections around the country and abroad. Once you find where primary sources are located, you are halfway there.

Covering Costs

The pursuit of any research will entail cost that should be taken into consideration and may be considerable. Expenses associated with joining the AAHN and attending conferences that require travel, food, and lodging all add to the cost of doing research. Purchasing books, traveling to archives, purchasing recording equipment to facilitate oral history recordings, and the transcription of those interviews can add up. When identifying primary sources, see what you find closer to home to help mitigate the cost of travel to far off locations. Although many archivists will send you copies of materials for a fee, that fee will be considerably less than the cost of travel to the site. One caveat here to keep in mind is that you do not want to limit yourself to one geographical location either.

Purchasing used books from Amazon and Barnes & Noble also helps keep the costs down. Some of the books I purchased this way had interesting signatures or were from nursing school libraries; for example, my copy of *Cornerstone for Nursing Education* has what appears to be the signature of the author Teresa Christy. As for recording oral histories, I used my daughter's old iPod Mini with a microphone that I purchased online. The same can be done with an iPhone. I did my own transcription of the two oral histories that I recorded for my dissertation, but it was time consuming.

I was encouraged to apply for funding for my research and did so through the AAHN. The grant I received, titled the H31 Predoctoral Award, was designed to encourage and support graduate training and historical research at the masters and doctoral level, and it covered much of the costs I mentioned previously. The grant application process is available on the website; receiving funding from this organization, which is rife with seasoned nurse historians, was a thrill. It validated my topic and encouraged my writing.

In addition to the predoctoral grant I was awarded at the beginning of my dissertation work, I was again encouraged to apply with my completed dissertation in 2012 for an AAHN award. I submitted my completed dissertation for the Teresa E. Christy Award for Exemplary Historical Research and Writing and received the award at the annual AAHN meeting in the fall of 2012. This was not a monetary award but simply a recognition of my work, and it proved invaluable both at my work and at professional meetings. It is one thing to complete your dissertation according to the rules and regulations of your graduate program but quite another to have your research recognized by historians outside of the institution, and I was fortunate to receive such recognition.

Time Constraints

Every doctoral student wants to complete his or her dissertation in a timely fashion, and I was no exception. The extensive reading and searching for resources can be both intimidating and exhausting. My advice to students considering a historical topic is first and foremost keep plenty of notes on whatever you read. I used an annotated bibliography when I began my research and included everything I read, even if I did not think it would apply to my final work. I made lists of items like the multiple reports on the status of nursing, such as *Nursing and Nursing Education in the United States: Report of the Committee for the Study of Nursing Education* (Goldmark, 1984 [originally published in 1923]), *Nursing for the Future* (Brown, 1948), and others, as a way to keep track of the time frame and contexts in which these reports were written. When you are ready to sit and interpret your data, you can refer to the notes. Be sure to use the correct format for references required by your institution, as it is time consuming to look up a reference for want of a page or other item that you forgot to include. One important point to note here is that although your institution may require one style manual, such as the American Psychological Association (APA), keep in mind that historians often use and publish using Chicago Style, which requires the first name of the author. It is worth looking into computerized programs like Zotero or End Note or some other way that you can keep all the data you need for future publications.

I myself did not use either of these programs, mostly because I was unfamiliar with them. For those who have used them, it is worth the time spent learning to use the programs. That is in my plans for the future. Whatever method you choose, keeping track of all the references for your dissertation cannot be overstated as this is a huge job, one that requires organization, patience, and tenacity. Several times I found myself remembering what I thought was an important piece of data and spent hours trying to find the reference.

Clear communication with your committee members helps prevent misunderstandings that can result in delays. Agreeing on turnaround times for materials is essential, especially as you approach the intimidating dissertation defense day. Determining a date that is convenient for all members of your committee can be frustrating, and an unexpected leave of absence or overseas trip of a faculty member can seriously delay the timing of your defense and, thus, graduation. My chair and I met on a regular schedule and communicated a lot by e-mail. We met at least once a month at the beginning of the process, and then more often as needed when I was collecting data. We also went together to some conferences, and we talked about the process as well as the content. The chair provides the primary critique of your work, and only after your chair and you are ready to send drafts does it go to the second reader on your committee. This is not true of all dissertation committees. You need to work within your organizational framework as each school will have its own protocol. Some have more seminars related to your topic, and those schools that have more historians on faculty like the University of Pennsylvania, may hold seminars where students can present their work and receive a critique from the larger group. You need to figure out your institution's dissertation protocols and work within these constraints, keeping focused and not getting discouraged.

Knowing When to Stop

Historical research lends itself to the so-called never-ending story and, indeed, it is never ending. But there is some point at which data collection must stop, and the interpretation of that data and the writing must begin. Rely on your committee members to guide you. I found the need to keep searching for more sources almost obsessive; had my committee members not stopped me, I may very well have not completed my dissertation. Lewenson's own experience with historian Nettie Birnbach telling her it was time to stop her data collection clearly influenced her advice to me that I had collected enough data at this point. And, in fact, Lewenson was right; it was not my life's work, and it was good enough to fulfill the requirements of my doctoral degree.

The completion of the dissertation is really just the beginning of the nurse historian's research. I think all historians feel that they are missing that one glaring tidbit of data that will answer all the questions. But this is the uncertainty and ambiguity of historical research. You will never find it all, and if you do, it may not be for your dissertation. The balance that you will struggle with is finding sufficient data that supports your research questions but does not extend the process into your twilight years. It is a difficult balance to find, and yet this is part of learning the historical method.

LESSONS LEARNED

Talk, talk, talk, and listen to your colleagues and faculty. Make the time to have dinner, drinks, lunch, and social connections, which is hard to do in this day and age, yet may lead to valuable "aha" moments. Networking can be exhausting, but the rewards are great. When I was working on my dissertation, I received a call out of the blue from a woman who was a student of Mildred Montag's when she started the program at Adelphi. This woman had heard of my research from someone at Adelphi and wanted to share with me her memories of Montag, whom she referred to as "a great lady." I was surprised that she found me and happy to hear more about Montag from the perspective of one of her original students.

Another lesson learned is to check out technology and to see how it will support your data collection. Equally useful is the reminder to stay on task. Although you need to continually read throughout the process, stay focused on your topic. Even though you will often stray from your original idea—and that's fine—give yourself a timeline to explore other materials. When you do find something of interest (but not on target), you can take a digital shot of the material you want to read for a future time. Keep a list of other topics that you are interested in for future research and publications. Keeping on task is a huge lesson to be learned. I continually felt that, since I was not writing, I was not progressing. But my committee members kept saying it was not the time to write but to read. And when it was time to write, I still read and wrote.

Choosing a Title

Although I had a working title throughout the process, one that changed multiple times, I did not come up with the final title until after the dissertation was just about finished. Among the points to keep in mind is a Google search. You want a title that people will find when they search the Internet for your topic. For instance, although I like the McManus quote used at the beginning of this chapter, "Pioneering requires imagination and foresight" (McManus to Arnold, January 9, 1953, p. 3), it really says nothing about my dissertation topic. So if anyone was doing an Internet search about the associate degree education for nurses or Mildred Montag or TC, it would not bring up any of my research. So, keeping this in mind, the title must include your topic and the years that you are looking at; even if it may not be the snappy title you want, it will get your work out there. My final title was *R. Louise McManus and Mildred Montag Create the Associate Degree Model for the Education of Nurses: The Right Leaders, the Right Time, the Right Place: 1947 to 1959*. It works as a dissertation title, but as I continue on with this topic, the title will change to reflect the direction of the research at that time.

NEXT STEPS

The completion of the dissertation represents a milestone in the life of the doctoral student. The graduate is now considered an expert in his or her field. Dissemination of the work is an important component of postdoctoral work and should include the presentation of materials at scholarly conferences and the submission of articles to peer review journals. Taking advantage of opportunities to be a guest lecturer and speak about the importance of the history of our profession is not only good experience for the newly minted doctor but informative for the students as well, given the dearth of history in the nursing curriculum. In my doctoral experience I formed close friendships with several colleagues, none of whom were doing historical research, yet each of whom provided valuable feedback to me throughout the dissertation process. I continue to meet yearly with them where we do informal roundtable discussions regarding our research interests and trajectory. We each have a list of items we want to accomplish, and every year we review and update our goals. In this way we stay connected and forward thinking. Our dissertations are not collecting dust, as some antiques do, but rather are the basis for our future publications and research. The nursing profession does not publish enough research, in particular historical research, because we do not socialize enough. Perhaps this can be a topic for yet another historical study.

My desire to learn a new method of research was the result of a combination of events. But as Gaddis (2002) posited:

> Studying the past is no sure guide to predicting the future. What it does do, though, is to prepare you for the future by expanding experience, so that you can increase your skills, your stamina—and, if all goes well, your wisdom. (p. 11)

I know I have the stamina and skills to "do" historical research and my journey certainly did expand my experience. For students considering a foray into historical research, I hope my experiences help expand your experience, as the nursing profession will be all the better for it.

REFERENCES

65 years of caring: The past and future of Adelphi's nursing program. (2009). *Illuminations: Newsletter from the school of nursing.* Retrieved from http://nursing.adelphi.edu/files/2013/05/illuminations_f09.pdf

American Nurses Association. (1965). American Nurses Association's first position paper on education for nursing. *American Journal of Nursing, 65*(12), 106–111.

Boschma, G. (2009). Sharing and presenting international nursing history research. *Nursing Inquiry, 16*(2), 93.

Brown, E. L. (1948). *Nursing for the future: A report prepared for the National Nursing Council.* New York, NY: Russell Sage Foundation.

Callaway, B. J. (2002). *Hildegard Peplau: Psychiatric nurse of the century.* New York, NY: Springer.

Champagne, M. T. (1981). *Innovation in nurse education: A history of the associate degree program, 1940–1964* (Unpublished doctoral dissertation). University of Texas, Austin, TX.

Christy, T. E. (1969). *Cornerstone for nursing education.* New York, NY: Teachers College Press.

Gaddis, J. L. (2002). *The landscape of history: How historians map the past.* New York, NY: Oxford University Press.

Goldmark, J. (1984). *Nursing and nursing education in the United States: Report of the committee for the study of nursing education.* New York, NY: Garland Publishing (Original work published 1923).

Lewenson, S. B., & Herrmann, E. K. (2008). *Capturing nursing history: A guide to historical methods in research.* New York, NY: Springer.

McAllister, A. (2012). *R. Louise McManus and Mildred Montag create the associate degree model for the education of nurses: The right leaders, the right time, the right place: 1947 to 1959* (Unpublished doctoral dissertation). Teachers College, Columbia University, New York, NY.

McManus to Arnold. (1953, January). Rockefeller Archive, RF collection, Record Group 1.2, Series 200, Box 166, Folder 1509. Rockefeller Foundation Archives, Rockefeller Archive Center, Pocantico, NY.

Montag, M. L. (1950). *Education of nursing technicians: A report of a type B project* (Unpublished doctoral dissertation). Teachers College, Columbia University, New York, NY.

Montag, M. L. (1951). *The education of nursing technicians.* New York, NY: Putnam.

Montag, M. L. (1959). *Community college education for nursing: An experiment in technical education for nursing.* New York, NY: McGraw-Hill.

President's Commission on Higher Education. (1946). *Higher education for American democracy.* New York, NY: Harper.

Safier, G. (1977). *Contemporary American leaders in nursing: An oral history.* New York, NY: McGraw-Hill.

Schorr, T. M., & Zimmerman, A. (1988). *Making choices, taking chances: Nurse leaders tell their stories.* St. Louis, MO: Mosby.

Euro-Pacific Film & Video Productions (Producer). (1999). *AD nursing: Revisiting our radical beginnings* [VHS]. Philadelphia, PA: Community College of Philadelphia.

CHAPTER FOUR

HISTORY IN THE MAKING: ORGANIZING A NURSING HISTORY DISSERTATION

Jeannine Uribe

This dissertation examines the interaction of U.S. and Chilean nurses, their governments, and the Rockefeller Foundation during a period of change in Chile's governmental responsibility for the welfare of their citizens. Trained nurse education began in Chile in 1902 under the guidance of physicians with ideas based on European nursing. Political changes in 1925 held the government responsible for state-sponsored programs, which included public health and sanitation, to better the health of all Chileans. Opening up a middle class bureaucracy, U.S. public health officials helped formulate policies and employment positions for the Chileans, and U.S. public health nursing was introduced in 1927. Chilean nurses built their profession by slowly increasing the number of schools, but the number of nurses grew slowly, and training and employment remained under physician control. A new presidential administration invited the Rockefeller Foundation to assist Chile in building their public health and nursing systems in 1941. Chilean nurses were given scholarships to study in U.S. and Canadian colleges to learn public health, administration, and education trends to build their profession. The study questions examined are: (a) Did the work of public health nurses change with each new presidential administration elected into office between 1927 and 1945? (b) Did the Rockefeller Foundation nurse consultants propose a program of nursing service that would radically transform public health practice in Chile? (c) Did U.S. influence transform the professional status of nurses and their role in the health care system of Chile? Chilean primary documents from the Biblioteca Nacional de Chile and U.S. Rockefeller Foundation documents were examined. Chilean nurses, with encouragement/ideas from the Rockefeller nurses, established public health nursing as an effective method for translating science to families to improve health and decrease morbidity and mortality. During this period, Chilean nurses gradually increased their control over the profession, strengthening their professional organization, increasing the number of nurse administrators, and fortifying their education system.

INTRODUCTION TO A HISTORICAL DISSERTATION

Health care changes rapidly with advancements in technology, communication, medications, and genetics. Nurses, the largest group of professionals in health, deal with the inflow of new ideas and continue to develop new policies, procedures, and skills to adapt and move forward. Nurse educators adapt curriculums to train nursing professionals to meet the hospital market's demands for competent workers. Few think about "why" nurses do what they do or how the hospital systems have been set up. The public and professionals alike live in current times without analysis of how we got into the situation we are in. Often, looking at the past shows the patterns and influences that created the trends we work under today. This is the importance of asking historical questions and completing historical research: How can we avoid cyclical patterns to make the best decisions for nursing?

Writing a doctoral dissertation in history is a solitary process. You do not have a research team that you are meeting with to teach protocol, discuss methodology, and review statistics. Research assistants, who gather your data and articles, are not part of the picture for this type of research. Your time will be spent with old documents in quiet archives and libraries, whispering your document requests to the archivists and librarians, who are ever helpful but do not have time to chat. You will be left alone with your thoughts and fears, questioning where each book and document fits into the big picture of your analysis. However, when you read the words of the people who have passed, realize the impact of their work, and see how events play out, you will be hooked, and you will find the determination to continue to uncover, analyze, and then write a historical dissertation. This chapter is meant to help you understand parts of the process and help smooth the way, so you can share your work with professionals and those interested in nursing history.

Historical research of the nursing profession comes under the umbrella of qualitative research, even though some historical works do include sections that are quantitative analyses; typically, nursing history is the analysis of leaders, events, and influences that shaped the nursing profession in its education, skills, work, management, licensure, policies, and other areas that make up the body of the profession. This chapter explains common experiences in completing a historical analysis for a nursing history dissertation as well as themes to help in the organization of your work.

FORMULATING IDEAS FOR A DISSERTATION TOPIC

Dissertation ideas often start from a doctoral student's point of knowledge of a subject or an experience that raises the question of inquiry to be investigated. It is recommended that you study a subject you feel passionate about or something that can hold your interest because you will deal with the topic, and topics that are connected to it, throughout the university writing years, as well as scholarly presentations and articles that will spin off from the dissertation.

Unlike students from the history department who have been students for many years and most likely do not have a professional background, nursing doctoral students of history have many years of experience in areas of nursing and have observed clients, nurses, managers, policies, and institutional systems that raise many questions. Working within health care systems and under policies that have political influences and nuances gives nursing doctoral students, who are now educated to think at a higher analytical level, new insight to consider the factors of how decisions have been made and how nursing arrived at its current state. With guidance and time, you can begin to formulate questions to investigate the historical context and actions to understand how nursing arrived at its current position.

Doctoral students often begin by taking on a large topic, unaware of the background investigation that is required to complete the dissertation. When thinking of an area to research, remember that the dissertation is only the opening paper of your future as a scholarly writer of history and to what can be discovered. It must be manageable for the time you have for the dissertation. The graduate group of your university does not want you to remain past the dates of expectation for finishing a dissertation. They want you to finish and emerge to become a productive nurse.

My first attempt to choose a topic of interest, when I approached the history group in the Barbara Bates Center for the Study of Nursing History at the University of Pennsylvania, was to study the U.S. Peace Corps nurses, a group of professionals sent out to the first selection of countries. Having spent 2 years in Paraguay as a Peace Corps volunteer rural health nurse from 1983 to 1985, I reflected now (20 years later) on the Peace Corps as a topic to research. History is not just a chronology of what took place but requires consideration of themes, consequences, context, and the players involved. Talking with faculty, I began to sift through my ideas to think of themes: What was accomplished by having Peace Corps nurses present? What did Peace Corps nurses bring to a country? How did they interact with the other professionals who were there? How did the Peace Corps goals coincide with the goals of the country's ministry of health? Being in the field and experiencing how the people lived their lives, did Peace Corps nurses carry out top-down goals or did they work with the community to complete grassroots goals? These questions attempt to examine the work of the nurses much more deeply than a historiography would.

Contemporary nursing events are valid as study subjects for a history dissertation; however, the faculty encouraged me to step back to another era to look at other situations when nurses were sent to foreign countries to work. Leaving mission work aside because of its religious connection and separate goals and focus, I was guided to look at nurses who worked in international philanthropies before the Peace Corps era. It is important to consider the primary sources available to examine alongside of developing a topic. Nurses have been viewed as small players in many institutions, so nursing documents may be difficult to find. Documents related to nurses and nursing actions have been archived, and it is helpful to write to archivists to ask about their collections and the documents that are listed in their "finding guides." Save time and worry by finding primary sources while developing the topic rather than finding out later that no evidence exists regarding your interest.

The faculty pointed me to the Rockefeller Archives in New York, an excellent archive because of their extensive documentation. The location of the archive, just 3 hours' drive from my home, meant I could schedule visits and arrive there in 1 day's travel. The archive contains diaries of their employees, telegrams, ticket stubs, yearly reports, and other correspondence with those outside of the organization. The International Health Division, the philanthropy started in the early 1900s by John D. Rockefeller, employed nurses and sent them to foreign countries to carry out a variety of nursing and health programs. Because of my experience in South America, I began to formulate my research questions based on the foundation's work to improve public health and to develop a public health nursing program in Chile in the 1940s.

Getting Organized

One of the first things to do is establish a documentation system to keep track of the many research notes, resources, and papers that are required for the doctoral degree and the dissertation. Organization cuts down on frustration and wasted time. Being able to find a document, an idea, or an article is critical for writing a history dissertation. Critical to understanding a topic you will include in your analysis is extensive reading, and keeping track of supporting ideas from other authors gives more depth to the dissertation. Locating the material right away saves time, keeps your writing flowing, and can prevent emotional breakdowns that occur in the stress of completing the dissertation.

First, organize all resources used. There are many great primary and secondary resources, so jump in and start reading and taking notes. Read books that relate to the topic, the time period, the politics, the economics, and other similar themes. Look in old newspapers and magazines for items that are related to the era or event, including people who were prominent during this time. This requires taking notes and filing items in a manner that allows one to find them again when wanting to write about a topic or section. Immersion through reading is an excellent way to get a perspective of the time period, even prior to establishing research questions. Reading to formulate the research questions of the dissertation proposal requires primary and secondary sources related to sections of the proposed questions.

In my dissertation, there were three large areas that I needed to investigate: public health nursing, the Rockefeller Foundation, and Chile. I needed to know about public health nursing, so I began to read books, analyzing the urban and rural work of U.S. public health nurses, their educational requirements, their clinical work, their professional organizations, and their leaders. I needed to have background knowledge of the Rockefeller Foundation's International Health Division, analyzed in biographies and in books that examined their philanthropic work not only in the United States but also in other countries, especially in Central and South America. A ministry of health is the health branch of a country's government, and so I read about the history of Chilean politics and political goals. I was also guided by the courses I studied during my second year of doctoral studies, each course chosen to provide historical analysis and other background information. All of these sources were tracked and recorded for future reference.

Using a calendar to organize is also very important for keeping track of meetings, seminar dates, payments, and other submissions for grants. Lay out a calendar for the year and keep it on a wall so you are aware of timelines for various requirements. It is easy to schedule on electronic gadgets, but it is harder to understand the overall picture of when things are due. Keeping timelines helps to prevent rushing to finish a requirement and allows prioritization.

I received two very important recommendations, and I continue to tell my friends who are going for their doctorate to do these two things, despite the abundance of technology. One is to buy a manila folder–sized portable file box for keeping records and copies of articles and pages that need to be copied onto paper, and two is to keep note cards. There are various systems to help you organize all the sources, so look into them and find the system that you understand and trust. You must also be aware of the licensing of each product: Can you take the information with you after graduation or do the references stay on the university's system? And be aware of the vulnerabilities: Does the system crash? How are improvements handled? One free electronic system, Zotero, allows you to keep track of sources and make notes. It can also import electronic reference information in the citation format of your choice. I was more comfortable using paper cards, so I set up my cards using 5 × 7 lined index cards and keeping a format: keywords in red in the upper right corner, citation on the left, important notes with page numbers and what were direct quotes—this is very important for avoiding plagiarism—underneath. I then used dividers to keep major keywords divided such as Rockefeller Foundation, U.S. public health nurses, Chilean politics, Chilean health care, and so on. It pays to talk to other students and to committee members to learn about different systems and to find the best fit.

Know your style of working. If you do not know, take one of the personality tests that can help you to recognize how you function to complete projects and how stress affects you. Are you ultra-organized and detail oriented? Consider whether your style matches your chair's so you can adapt to her or his style and prevent derision. Are you a procrastinator who will be extremely stressed in the week before a chapter is due and fall apart if the schedule is moved up? The logistics of finishing a doctoral dissertation depend upon the doctoral student's drive to complete a dissertation. Classwork, while challenging, guides the student with a syllabus, assignment due dates, course meetings, and deadlines that are not formulated for your dissertation work. Realizing you are ultimately the only one responsible for how much you have written is stressful and can be overwhelming, leading to cantankerous behavior that can tarnish relationships. The dissertation becomes the guiding force of your life, and you must be mature enough to plan your life to get it done. You must be aware of this and be patient with yourself but continue to strive to better your work habits and to set deadlines, even if you have always been a procrastinator. Thank those friends and family who are helping you and trying to allow you the space to write; they do not understand the process and just want to assist you. In the end, organization and fortitude are what will help you get to the defense of your dissertation.

Choosing a Committee for a History Dissertation

Choosing your chair and your committee is a very important activity, which starts when you are applying to a school. You want to choose a school with faculty who are comfortable working with a history dissertation or, at the very least, are well versed in your topic of interest so that they can guide you and include examples and discussions of their own work. Your work may be part of the gap in knowledge of the work they are doing, so it is beneficial to know the faculty and their work when applying. Of course, it is a luxury if you have the freedom to apply to a variety of schools and to move to be near the university where you are accepted, but it is usually not practical. Online doctoral programs can offer you the ability to complete your doctorate with annual or occasional meetings on campus. Just be sure to ask about doing a history dissertation and investigate the history department professors and their articles and published books.

Many committee chairs are well-known researchers with years of work and national reputations. They are very busy lecturing, teaching, and researching, which is one of the reasons why you choose them. You must respect their time and plan meetings well in advance to avoid having them rush through meetings and your chapters. Ask them how they prefer to see your work. Maybe they work better with a paper copy so they can write on it and give it back to you. If they are traveling, maybe they prefer a digital copy, which is properly formatted and in a 12-point font so they can easily read it on an airplane. Make friends with the chair's administrative assistant, who will let you know your chair's schedule of meetings and vacations as well as other things about him or her. The assistant can become your ally, letting you know the secrets of how to work best with your chair.

You must be respectful of your chair's time, which is a fine line to navigate. Given too much time, a busy researcher may put your chapter aside to read later and then forget it. Given too little time, a chair may develop a stressful situation with only time to give your work a glance. When interviewing with your chair and making the agreement, ask these important questions about working together: How is it best to contact him or her? Does the chair want a weekly or a monthly meeting? Who arranges that? Is the chair available on phone? Is e-mail best? Things can become buried in e-mails because of the large number of mails faculty receive, so ask which method is the best way to stay in touch. Try to set deadlines so that your chair is also aware of how you work and when your items are due.

Many universities with colleges of nursing also have a history department, and you will want to consider the work they are doing as well because faculty from other colleges in the university add depth to your knowledge and richness to your writing. Completing a history dissertation in a nursing department without a nurse historian as faculty is more challenging but not unworkable because many things about history are different. Many researchers use APA formatting and citations, whereas historians use Chicago Style citations. Pulling together history chapters is very different from laying out a typical quantitative dissertation with standard headings often seen in published studies. Your chair needs to be in support of your historical research or at least willing to assist you in learning about the process. If you feel you are being pushed into a different pathway and that this chair may not support your history interest, you may delay writing because you are trying to convince them of the importance of your work.

Asking a history faculty member is also very important even though he or she will not be your chairperson. The history faculty members will be knowledgeable in historical analysis and writing and can help guide you to important works on the topic. It is expected that you will take courses related to historical analysis, working with documents, critiquing secondary sources, and other history courses on your doctoral program. You will take the core courses related to doctoral-level thinking in nursing, research, statistics, and other core courses for a nursing doctorate, but the next courses are related to your topic. Remember, you are expected to be an expert in your topic by the time your dissertation is finished and to have developed skills for analyzing history.

My steepest learning curve was with readings in Chilean history, not only related to their history of health care but also their formation as a state, their politics, and their relationship with the United States. Chilean nursing history was very difficult to find because of the lack of published papers on the subject and lack of digitalized documents. My chair guided me to choose a professor in Latin American history who could direct me to readings and writings on Chilean history to understand the country from a Latin American studies perspective. Dr. Farnsworth-Alvear's knowledge helped me to understand and analyze Chile from a social history framework. Without her guidance, my dissertation would have been superficial in terms of Chilean history. The following is an extract from my dissertation:

> The image of nurse as assistant to a physician limited the autonomy of the nurse leaders and placed them in a position they did not alter. In her book on Colombian factory workers, Farnsworth-Alvear points out that the factory women earned their social status from the rules imposed by their employers and had to conform to their ideas of the

"norms of respectable femininity." Nursing in Chile had rules and social norms imposed upon them based on their gender, their work, and expectations for both. Pincheira's desire to take charge of the school of nursing came from outside of the culture, from the United States, and had her acting outside of the traditional, conservative, feminine role of nurse–mother and physician–assistant, the role the nurse held by the physician's side. The paternal medical system responded by taking away nursing's ability to manage itself and placed a physician in charge with a committee of physicians to watch over the school. Some physicians tried to downgrade the high educational requirement for entrance to training, a move that would have placed nursing in a more subservient status. Social workers, free from the domestic role attached to nursing and outside of the realm of the physician, were able to manage themselves, and even though they did not receive the university diploma, they earned higher salaries and held a higher interest for young women. (Uribe, 2008, pp. 88–89)

The process of obtaining a doctorate may vary with each university, but typically you will need to pass the steps before getting to the dissertation seminar where you begin to formulate your dissertation proposal. Successful completion of comps, qualifying exam, and other writing on methodology gives the student the background knowledge on the topic and shows the chair the student's ability to think critically about history and to write cohesively.

During the dissertation seminar, where your cohort comes together to discuss and justify proposal ideas and give valuable feedback, you may again need to explain your historical research. Take every opportunity to present well and answer questions, being honest if you do not know the answer but then going to look up the answer or discuss the answer with your mentors. You need to take every opportunity to put into words just what you are doing. This is the time to reformulate your question and fine tune your topics. Your cohort will help you to rationalize and focus your topic because they do not know much about the history you are writing. Listen to their questions and answer them, but also realize they might not know the historical analysis process; therefore, this is a great time to establish your thinking on the topic. Explaining what you are doing always helps to fine tune your message and to realize just what you need to learn about to carry out your work.

During my dissertation seminar, I had been writing my proposal (the layout of my research argument) about the Rockefeller work in South America, and I was in love with Argentina and its people. I wrote up my proposal saying I would investigate the work of the Rockefeller Foundation in Argentina as the basis for my work. The night before I was to present in class, I came across an online finding guide to the papers at the Rockefeller Archive and compared the cubic foot size of the boxes of files for each country in South America. Colombia had a large collection as did Chile. Argentina had very little listed. The next morning, while explaining my proposal to the class of probably 10 quantitative student researchers and three qualitative researchers, I changed the country to Chile, knowing there were more folders documenting the work in Chile than in Argentina. Everyone laughed and went along with it, understanding the lack of discernment at this stage of one's research. Later, I found out that Santiago, Chile, was the headquarters of the Rockefeller Foundation's work in the Southern Cone and realized I had made the right decision. If I had not changed my mind at that point, my first visit to the archives would have told me that there was not much in terms of work in Argentina, and my proposal would have to be officially changed, wasting time. The following is an extract from my dissertation:

> Hackett decided that Brackett needed to remain in Santiago to assist in the set up of the first unidad sanitaria (health units). This was to be a large, mutual project between the agency and the Chilean government with financial contributions shared by both institutions. It would be the model health unit used for patient care and as a training center for public health nurses and physicians. Brackett arrived in Santiago on July 17, 1942, checking into the finest hotel in the city, and headed out to the IHD offices to meet the Chilean staff and Dr. John H. Janney, a U.S. physician in charge of the Chilean programs. (Uribe, 2008, p. 140)

Travel Grants and Funding

Living the life of a doctoral student can be economically stressful because of the decreased income, added expenses for books, and other expenses that arise. History research has its own expenses. Traveling to archives can be expensive once you consider overnight stays, spending for gas, air fare, and parking. Meals need to be taken into consideration; alternatively, brown bagging may be necessary, as some archives are isolated without restaurants nearby. It is very important to figure out how to get to the archive before leaving. Does the archive provide transportation between train lines and the archive? Is it walkable from the train stop? Can the staff recommend hotels that are not far? As the Internet has grown, so has the ease of planning to visit archives.

During your visit, you may be assigned an archivist who is familiar with the records you want to research. This is a person who understands the structure of the archives and how information is stored. This person can also investigate other areas that may be connected to your work. For my visit to the Rockefeller Archive, there were files for the health office in Santiago giving information on the personnel. There were also other files in a human resources section that contained the background of the U.S. nurses, which allowed me to understand their educational background and the area where they grew up. The archivist also suggested I look at the files of annual reports that summarized the year's activities, substantiating dates and information in the other documents, letters, and diaries.

Some of the larger archives may offer travel grants to help you to get to the archive. You can find these online or by making a phone call to see how and when to apply. Copying costs, travel expenses, and hotel costs are allowed to be covered in the budget you prepare and must be used toward visiting the archive. After your research, the archive grant will require you to write up a short article on what you found. This is not a research article but rather discusses what material is present and why you wanted to look at it for your research topic.

Planning your visit in advance is important to allow you to arrive on the dates you want to visit the archive. Some archives are very busy with foreign visitors in the summer and their research slots fill up, so lay out your schedule. Other archives do not have as many visitors and will allow you to give just a few days' notice before coming. This notice allows them to pull the requested information for you so it is ready when you arrive. At the end of your time at the archive or at the end of the day, let the archivist know which materials you want copied, which you are finished with, and whether or not you are returning the next day. Typically, they will keep your materials together for you for the next day. Or, if you are finished, they can place them back in their spot. This again allows you to use your time in the best manner.

Each archive has its own system of providing documents to you. There may be restrictions on the material you are examining, depending upon the rules of the archive. For my dissertation, the Presbyterian Historical Society in Philadelphia held the papers and letters of the Presbyterian missionary nurses who worked in Chile in the 1930s. Their website directed me to write a letter of intent to the archive, describing the papers I wanted to look at and the dates of the papers. I was granted a very specific window during which I could examine them. Their rules support the privacy of members still living. One of the missionary nurses was still alive, so I could not use her papers; however, the papers of the nurses who had passed away were available to be examined.

You may be allowed to photograph items with your own camera. However, you may need to pay for copies, and these copies may be sent to you at a later date. Copying archival documents is expensive and takes time. Currently, some archives allow different methods for copying data. Handheld scanners are helpful, as are photographs. You must have the permission of the archive to use this equipment, and they will be very clear with you about what is allowed. You must also be aware of the copyrights of the material for use in future presentations and publications. Permission may be required for use of pictures in your thesis. Keep copies of the papers you sign when using the archive.

Archive Considerations

Internet searching gives the student access to archives, helps in finding aids, and leads to information. Finding aids tell the researcher overall categories for information that may be found on the person, topic, country, and a variety of other search words. A variety of ways exist to search for a person. For nurses, uncovering their training school and looking at their application can give the researcher information such as home town, health, religion, and how their professors viewed them in school, including hours completed in training, days absent, and their predilection for areas of nursing.

To understand the background of the nurses who went to Chile with the Rockefeller Foundation, I looked into documents that uncovered many interesting items about their backgrounds, their past employers, and their passing. Looking at past employers revealed connections that referred Mary Elizabeth Tennant to the Rockefeller Foundation. The following is an extract from my dissertation:

> To understand the analysis and importance placed on policies and activities held dear to the public health nurse consultants, one can examine the backgrounds and writings of the people responsible for choosing the criteria to be analyzed in the curriculum and practice of Chilean nursing. The nursing section of the RF raised leaders who continued to do innovative projects or teach after leaving the Foundation. (Uribe, 2008, pp. 111–113)

The Rockefeller Foundation's Nurse Leader

The Rockefeller Foundation chose U.S. nursing staff with years of experience and expertise in their fields to train the future leaders of other countries. Mary Elizabeth Tennant was the nurse in charge of the IHD's nursing programs, and she traveled all over the world for more than 20 years analyzing and setting up public health nursing programs. Born in Colorado, Mary Elizabeth Tennant was honored in her small high school as a basketball player and as the head of the athletics club in 1912 (Wahatoya, 1912). She was well educated, starting with her graduation from the University of Colorado with a bachelor's degree in teaching. With her degree, Tennant became the principal of a public school in Tollerburg, Colorado, for 2 years. What drew her to change careers and go to the Vassar College training camp for nurses in 1918 may have been what attracted many young college-educated women—the patriotic desire to serve their country during a nursing shortage (Dreves, 1975). The training camp candidates had to be college educated because "their previous education facilitates intensive training and more rapid advancement to posts of urgent need" (Clappison, 1964, p. 18). Graduating from the 11-week summer camp where they practiced the "three principles that nurses need to develop: promptness, regularity, and habits of obedience" (Clappison, 1964, p. 19), she entered nurses' training at Philadelphia General Hospital, finishing as planned in 2 years and 3 months (Clappison, 1964, p. 19). In Pennsylvania, she studied hospital duties and procedures, taking classes and working the hospital floors as a student until she received her diploma in 1920. The camp promoted the duties and the need for public health nurses; therefore, after basic hospital training, she continued her education and interest in public health at Simmons College in Boston by taking public health nursing courses. She gained the notation BSc (bachelor of science) after her name as well as PHN (public health nurse) from her 1 year at Simmons. Her foundation résumé also lists attendance at Harvard Medical College from 1920 to 1921, which at one point combined with Simmons College to offer a school for social workers, covering many topics aimed at social service, so she may have taken social work courses through Harvard ("School for Social Workers," 1905).

With a solid education in public health nursing, Tennant returned home to her native Colorado to become the assistant superintendent of the Denver Visiting Nurse Association, gaining nursing and supervisory experience and then seeking another supervisory position nearby. After only 1 year, she moved on to become the supervisor of school nursing for the Denver public school system, which lasted only 3 months before she was off to New York to become the field supervisor of the Nursing Welfare Division of the Metropolitan Life Insurance Company (MLIC), perhaps recommended for the position by the connections she made in the Vassar summer camp.

The MLIC sent public health nurses to visit the homes of families insured by their company. It was an idea put forth by Lillian Wald promoting nursing with evidence of nurses assisting to better the health of the policy holders. Her work as field supervisor of the visiting nurses put her in close contact with the Henry Street Settlement administration, a settlement house established in 1893 to work with the Eastern European immigrants, who were arriving in large numbers. The settlement was also a training ground for public health nurses coming from all parts of the United States and some foreign countries, who then went home with genuine clinical experience in public health nursing. With this training under their belts, they returned to their jobs better able to function in their positions. The Henry Street Settlement became the site for the international Rockefeller fellows to gain home visiting experience during their training in the United States (Uribe, 2008, pp. 111–113).

Confirming information is an important part of vetting the documents one will use for history. Congruency is achieved by following up on information threads and then connecting the links. For my dissertation, a general Internet search for Mary Elizabeth Tennant opened up a document of her high school yearbook in Colorado, showing her leadership on the basketball court and her future in teaching. She received her teaching degree and then decided to join the patriotic movement of the Vassar Training Camp for Nurses in 1918 to become a nurse. She applied to Philadelphia General Hospital (PGH). Records for PGH are archived in Philadelphia, so I viewed her PGH application that confirmed the town she was in and the high school she attended. The Internet information, a digital picture in the yearbook, is now confirmed to be the Mary Elizabeth Tennant of the Rockefeller Foundation. Other notes found in her PGH file confirm her work in the foundation because she wrote to the head of the school, Lillian Clayton, regarding what she was doing after graduation.

Contacting the archive to understand their finding aids, their documents, their hours of operation, and their rules is important before traveling. Government archives are closed on major holidays. Private archives may or may not be. Arriving early may be important if the archives fill up on a first come first served basis. It is also important to notify the archive so that your documents are pulled and prepared for your arrival so that you can get started in your search when you get there. Of course, that is if the archive allows you to schedule a visit. Many archivists know the collections or will investigate further for you; therefore, if there is a "contact us" portion, you may approach it to ensure the archive holds the information you want to review. When political papers are involved, you want to know what is in what archive because presidential archives can hold papers connected to presidential administrations.

CHAPTER 4. ORGANIZING A NURSING HISTORY DISSERTATION   73

Corroborating the Evidence

Diaries can lead to many new discoveries and can branch out to include information that can add to understanding the context of the times and the situation in the country. Brackett's Rockefeller diary listed her daily activities and her meetings. She mentioned her encounters with nurses from the Presbyterian mission group. With those names, I was able to search the archives of the Presbyterian Church in Philadelphia. While I had to be careful to avoid going off too deeply into the branch of missionary nursing, I did find the mission nurses' letters interesting. The mission nurses were also trying to start nursing programs and they wrote home to their funders about the reasons their plans were delayed. Although the Church is also a philanthropic organization, the documents were used only to add to the understanding of the context of the time. Brackett was writing to the Rockefeller Foundation, addressing their needs, while the Presbyterian nurses were writing to their mission foundation to answer their inquiries. The observations of the missionary nurses in Chile corroborated the information Brackett wrote about by confirming the educational issues, cultural issues of women in society, as well as the status of nursing and government policy for nursing education.

Footnotes or Endnotes

Every doctoral student will come across people, events, or documents that add contextual information and are seemingly important and very interesting but are not significant for answering the research questions; they may also take the reader to a new point without answering the prior point. Typically, this is information that should be reserved for a footnote or endnote. The information adds to the understanding of the behind-the-scenes events or the background information of people involved but takes focus away from the analysis. The following is an extract from my dissertation:

> Auxiliary health workers were needed to introduce the prevention message to workers. Workers met with a physician and nurse during the mandatory physical exam screening for disease and may have heard tips on hygiene and disease prevention during the exam or while in the waiting room. They may have read the Ministry posters on the clinic walls on how to prevent the spread of disease or read government pamphlets. One of the Presbyterian missionary nurses commented on the value of the new social security laws saying, "...for with so many

benefits from the Social Security Laws, even the most ignorant people are beginning to lose their fear of hospitals, and are becoming more germ conscious as typhoid fever rages among them". Nurses who had studied the public health nursing course were taught the principles of preventive education, and there were professional discussions in the journals between physicians on education for mothers for prenatal care and newborn care. So, it is possible that patients that came in for their physical examination also got information from nurses and physicians on health prevention while in the clinic. Clinics also held weekly Mother's clubs with the intention of teaching mothers about care for themselves and their children and some domestic tasks related to nutritious meal planning and sewing clothing for the family. (Paden, R., 1934; Uribe, 2008, p. 96)

The footnote says: Rose Paden, Station Letter 19 October 1934, RG 160, Series 9, Box 4, Folder 25, Presbyterian Historical Society. Paden wrote station letters to report on her activities to the people who sent money to support her and who prayed for her mission. Paden wrote about the posters, pamphlets, and instructions given to mothers visiting the dispensary in Valparaiso. The literacy rate was increasing at the time but Paden's notes do not comment on whether the mothers could read the pamphlets or if the pamphlets had pictures. The government is known to have a health education department within the health department (Uribe, 2008, p. 96).

The footnote may also include information from other books that back up the statement you are making or help to explain your thinking in the analysis. The following is an extract from my dissertation:

> Prenatal care by midwives and physicians existed, though before Law 6174, many mothers sought prenatal care late in the pregnancy either exhibiting symptoms of a difficult pregnancy or ready to deliver (Frakia, 1943). Arriving to deliver a baby without prenatal care sometimes resulted in complications related to high blood pressure, anemia, and other unanticipated problems affecting the health of both mother and child.
>
> The malnutrition problem in Chile potentially increased both maternal and infant morbidity and mortality rates, before, during, and after birth. Although birth weight was not counted in the statistics in the 1930s and 1940s, it is now known that malnutrition affects the birth weight of the baby. Those babies weighing less than 2,500 grams at birth due to malnutrition most likely started life with the added burden of the other factors contributing to the high infant mortality in Chile.

The law proposed prenatal visits, birth attendance by physicians or registered midwives, and registration of the infant into the health system (Frakia, 1943). The midwives handling home births were particularly important in the registration process of infants introducing mothers to the need for frequent infant check-ups. The standardized, recommended schedule for infant visits depended on the infant's condition at birth requiring shorter intervals between visits for infants born with congenital defects, or those infants of mothers that had problems before or during birth (Frakia, 1943). Infant programs included infant weights, vaccinations, giving out milk, and checking for gastrointestinal and respiratory illnesses.

Part of Alessandri's economic recovery plan required raising taxes charged to foreigners in order to maintain the state bureaucracy and pacify workers (Monteón, 1998). The military, the police, and the education system took a large percentage of his budget yet his administration continued to plan programs to educate workers hoping to build nationalistic feelings. He created a Cultural Extension Department in the Ministry of Labor to give the workers culture through theater, books, lectures, and other means (Barr-Melej, 2001). His support for public health education remained small and underfunded because medicine remained the major focus in the health care.

Dr. Eduardo Cruz-Coke, Minister of Health in the Alessandri cabinet, assisted in the writing and promotion of the new health law in 1938. It was a step towards promoting social medicine, though Alessandri gained more support from Conservative and Liberal Party members and lost the support of the Radical Party (Monteón, 1998). The law was passed and enacted in spite of the length of time it would take to install and expand the clinic structure and train and hire the personnel needed to carry it out (de Ramón, 2001). The program's direction began within the Ministry of Health, which then passed the regulations to the administrators in each insurance caja. These managers then had the responsibility to fulfill the provisions of the law for their clientele, including the contracting of and the payment to physicians for the required, periodic physical examinations and tests. The administrator also distributed the payment to the disabled worker for the physician-determined, mandatory rest to prevent a worsening of disease or retirement in the case of advanced disease (Ley 6174, 1938). Inequalities were seen because each insurance caja interpreted the order differently and carried out its work on a different schedule delaying service to some areas of the country and some employment groups. Politics unevenly granted benefits to the different cajas resulting in differences between groups. (Collier & Sater, 2001; Uribe, 2008, pp. 93–95)

The footnotes in the original dissertation address an article written by a nurse and four books, as well as the Law 6174 from the Preventive Medicine book. Therefore, the explanations of the political parties was necessary for understanding further the political standings, but would have taken up a lot of room to explain within the paragraph.

Setting the Time Period

Setting the time period of your research is very important because you can continue to search for evidence, which will continue to reveal new information, and it will feel like you will never finish. Establishing a time period around the event or person you are studying helps you to limit your focus and to avoid looking at documents too far outside of that time period. An important mantra during the investigative period has to be, "This is my first work. That point is related but I will follow that lead after the dissertation." And those leads you determine to be outside of your time period can be mentioned in the last chapter of your dissertation, proposing further research you will complete.

The first timeline for my proposal centered on the Rockefeller time period in Chile, 1941 to 1952, when the IHD was active. The RF arrived in December 1941, as Pearl Harbor was being bombed. Tennant was actually in Santiago, Chile, on December 7, 1941, and noted in her diary she heard the U.S. declaration of war on the radio. I chose to end my period of analysis at 1945 because it is easily recognizable as the end of World War II, in terms of surrender, and the beginning of the reconstruction of Europe and Japan. The cutoff date was not set by the war but by the big changes accompanying the shift in economics and peacetime living. New systems and processes were established in health, and the Rockefeller Foundation's IHD refocused financial support to Europe while pulling it out of Latin American countries. The World Health Organization (WHO) gained importance in unifying health care information, consultation, and research, and the Pan American Sanitary Bureau (PASB), a regional arm of the WHO, hired nurses to consult with Latin American countries. These changes made the era the perfect time to set as the end of the period of analysis because the changes that occurred postwar took Chilean nursing in a different direction, which would have required a lot of investigation of the work of those new institutions.

Determination of the start of the time period also took consideration: where to begin the analysis. I started my research at the Rockefeller Archives, looking at what their nurses found. However, I did not have an explanation for why the profession was in the condition that it was. I felt it was important to understand how Chilean nursing started and what support it had from the educational and governmental institutions. One book was written by the head of the school of nursing in the University of Chile. It was a celebratory description of the history of nursing in Chile and showed several links to U.S. nursing. These links were important for me to understand how Chilean nurses felt toward U.S. nurses and our nursing system. I changed my time period based on the information in this book, knowing that I had to understand the connections or influences of U.S. nursing trends in Chilean nursing history. It was a much bigger task to begin my search when nurses first trained in Chile rather than starting with the nursing system in 1941, but it was critical for understanding. The British influence was present and a physician, Edward Moore, who is credited with starting nursing in 1902, visited Britain to investigate the Nightingale system. The following is an extract from my dissertation:

> The growing body of scientific, medical, and surgical knowledge used by physicians relieved suffering and illness in patients; however, a patient's return to health was not immediate, and physicians needed assistants to carry out procedures, give medicines, change dressings, and follow their orders until the patient no longer needed attention. As noted above, Dr. Eduardo Moore Bravo saw the value of a nurse to his practice of medicine as well as to the care of the sick in his country (Flores, 1965). He took a grand tour of Europe, specifically allotting time to observe and study medicine and the health care system of England and France. The nurses practicing in the hospitals under the "Nightingale system" caught his attention, and he brought back the idea of training lay women to nurse the sick (Lanza Lazcano, 1998). The instruction he set up revolved around a three-year course for nurses to begin at the Hospital San Francisco de Borja in the southern section of Santiago in 1902 (Laval, 1944). Twenty-eight graduates finished the first 3-year course in 1905, and the number of students admitted to study increased after that year. A majority of the women were recruited from middle class backgrounds with a higher level of education than the average woman in the country.
>
> Dr. Moore incorporated some educational policies into the nurses training that were similar to the university where he taught

medicine. The nursing studies lasted 3 years and were divided into six semesters with a test prepared by the professors at the end of each semester. Three hours of daily clinical studies on the hospital floor was expected in most classes, and Moore provided a list of 16 subjects that the students studied at least once and perhaps twice during their 3 years, naming classes on anatomy, physiology, internal medicine, obstetrics, physical therapy, chronic medicine, and a host of classes on the ethical and legal issues of Chilean medicine and nursing.

From the start, Dr. Moore introduced nursing as a lay, feminine profession to be placed under the watch of the physician and hired for his benefit. He offered the new profession of lay nursing as an honorable, vocational, and noble work, a vocational calling within women's natural propensity. The rules established for the first school required students to have "an irreproachable morality" and were meant to ease the public criticism from conservative citizens toward this traditionally pious work of nuns (Flores, 1965). The educational standard called for an elementary education, which was limited to girls because of the limited number of public schools and room for female students. Many of the girls educated above the fourth grade level were educated at home with tutors paid for by the family or attended private Catholic schools. Education was a privilege few but the well-to-do could afford. Chosen candidates conveyed the personal attributes of a "spirit of sacrifice," and "solid moral attributes" as well as a "love for the suffering humanity," qualities sounding very similar to a religious calling and very difficult to objectively quantify (Flores, 1965).

Using Flores' book to make a timeline, I found her narrative did contain documents to back up her observations. However, further documentation was needed, and a trip to Chile was planned to locate primary sources to give the Chilean viewpoint and to document their ideas of nursing, the politics related to nursing, and university documents. The librarians were helpful in pointing me to the university documents of published meetings and journals that contained editorials and newspaper clippings. Because of my limited time in the country, I paid for copies of all of the pages so I could translate and analyze them at home. I wanted to keep searching to find as much as I could in my 2 weeks. A last minute visit to the Chilean Nurses Association did not allow me to see primary source documents of the organization but did give some journal articles documenting activities in the 1960s written by the nurses who had worked with the Rockefeller Foundation nurses. This information was helpful in my summary and conclusions section and helped to formulate further work to be researched in the history of Chilean nursing. The following is an extract from my dissertation:

> Future studies are needed to examine how public health nurses responded to the dramatic changes that followed the time period of this study. An examination is needed of the reaction of the nursing leadership and funding as all nurses had to register in the face of a growing demand. All health organizations and institutions were placed under one ruling body, called the National Health Service, an idea that originated with Dr. Salvador Allende while he was Minister of Health. There was an increased need for public health nurses to fill positions in the growing state bureaucracy and nurses had the answers to the questions about their profession. Nursing professionalism grew as nurses gained leadership positions in education, management, and state organizations. The Chilean nurses joined the International Council of Nurses, a membership made possible by the formation of the College of Nurses of Chile that required all nurses to register before employment. (Uribe, 2008, pp. 212–213)

Justification for your time period choice is an important discussion to have with your chair and committee members so you are not overextending the period of analysis or missing an important event that may have an impact. You will have to validate your time period in the introduction, in the setting, in the summary, in the conclusions, and in its significance. In the beginning weeks of research, you are adjusting your understanding of the information, and thus the period may vary. However, it is important to consider this so you can focus your time.

Translating Documents

Finding documentation from another country and in another language gives the view of the other side and helps broaden the understanding of the historical time period, as well as helps to prevent bias in the analysis. Care must be taken to interpret the words carefully, and as with any source, one must consider the distinctiveness of the document: who wrote it, why it was written, for whom it was written, and what it says. This also becomes part of the thesis, showing your analysis.

In my dissertation, during the 1940s, Salvadore Allende, who had a political agenda, was a candidate for a congressional seat. He wrote a book, *La Realidad Médico-Social Chilena*. The following is an extract from my dissertation:

> Aguirre Cerda had no plans to stop the preventive health law already in place although his Minister of Health, a powerful Socialist party member, Dr. Salvador Allende, made new plans to augment and reorganize the state-run health care delivery system.
>
> Due to the successful resolution of the economic problems by the previous president, Aguirre Cerda came to power in a country that, although recovering economically with higher employment and increased trade, continued to be plagued by high morbidity and mortality rates concentrated among the working class and the poor. The return to national, fiscal stability meant the government had money to cover a budget and Dr. Salvador Allende, the Minister of Health, followed his Socialist beliefs of providing social welfare programs for the workers (Drake, 1973).
>
> Allende held strong Marxist, socialist beliefs, which permeated his medical work and health plan for the country. As minister and cabinet member, he researched the health needs of Chileans and published the results in a book [,] *La Realidad Médico-Social Chilena* [,] dissecting the health and welfare of the Chilean people and recommending solutions to the problems he foresaw as a result of economic underdevelopment related to dependence on foreign capital. Allende's book was radical and his view of social medicine differed from European views because of the connection and relationship of problems to foreign business. The Popular Front administration permitted Allende to implement his vision of social medicine and to make a plan to nationalize the health system, which was not implemented until 1952. (Allende, 1939).
>
> Allende took apart the necessities of life, breaking down the cost of food and housing and comparing it to salaries earned. Using the statistical research of others as well as studies he conducted, Allende broke down the caloric needs of workers, the cost of food, and salary earned discovering through mathematical calculation that Chilean workers did not meet their families' basic needs for food, and thus became ill more often from the lack of proper nutrition (Allende, 1939). He analyzed the statistics for food production and compared it to a normal consumption pointing out Chile's deficits in milk production and other foods (Allende, 1939). His statistics showed that little of the worker's money was left over at the end of the month because food accounted for 80%

of the worker's budget compared to a worker in the United States who used only 30.2% of the budget for food (Allende, 1939). Allende saw Chile's deficiencies as underdevelopment compared to the developed nations of Europe and the United States. (Uribe, 2008, pp. 101–103)

Translating aged documents into another language can create misunderstanding in the meaning of the words. Word usage changes over time and may not be understood. The definition of words in Spanish changes from country to country, so the doctoral student must be careful to interpret the words correctly. Institutional documents contain formal jargon as well as system and processing words that may not translate clearly. The following is an extract from my dissertation:

> The other piece of evidence regarding the limited number of nurses produced by Chile, attracting young women to the profession, became important to consider because public health nurses' work was not seen by the middle class nor were the home visiting nurses visiting their homes. The university decided to promote its nursing program to the isolated and slowly growing southern regions of Chile. With the only recognized nursing schools located in the middle and northern sections of the country, young women living in the south rarely applied. In order to drum up interest in the nursing profession and the schools, university representatives traveled to the outer regions of Chile to talk to students and present their university program. An ex-sub-director of the school, Nurse Teresa Hernandez, traveled with two other physicians in the school of nursing, to the beautiful lake region in the south and the big cities of Puerto Montt, Temuco, Chillián, Osorno, and Valdivia. Although the university representatives were gone for a short 7 days, two of which were spent traveling to the region, each stop accomplished the intended goal of exposing young women to the idea of entering the profession of nursing. They met with prospective 5th and 6th year humanidades students and those in the liceo (university prep school to prepare for the bachillerato exam) to promote the university educated profession of nursing. The tour received some press, publicized in the local newspapers as a feminine profession so that young women and their families learned of the many opportunities for work in the new "public mission" of nursing. (Uribe, 2008, pp. 77–78)

The *charlas* (small group presentations) spoke of the employment opportunities within the state bureaucracy working for a variety of hospitals, the workers insurance organizations, the welfare institutions, and the private duty sector. To bring more interest to the profession, this traveling group of university professors promoted nursing by advertising the new specialties of psychiatric and dietetic nursing that were being developed in other countries. Even with state sponsorship for a university nursing education and the promise of available jobs in the state bureaucracy, women failed to enter nursing, and a nursing shortage developed.

Unless one is fluent in a second language, translation of documents can be done by a certified translation service. If you have the knowledge of the language and want to attempt to do the translations yourself, one way to avoid issues is to provide the original language quotation as well as your translation of the quote in the same paragraph. This allows readers to translate the quote for themselves if they speak the language. For those who are not literate in that language, seeing the words in another language and then seeing the translation in English gives depth to their reading. The following is an extract from my dissertation:

> Flores' writing hints at some controversy surrounding Dr. Moore's nursing program by saying, "Serias dificultades amenazaron la feliz realizacion de esta iniciativa. Intereses creados y prejuicios religiosos, se hicieron presente ante la nueva y revolucionaria concepción de la enfermería laica y femenina" (Flores, 1965, p. 35). "Serious difficulties threatened the happy realization of this initiative. Created interests and religious prejudices have become present before the new and revolutionary concept of lay, feminine nursing" (Flores, 1965, p. 35). Social norms were at stake with a new profession for women. Honorable women of the higher levels of society did not work outside of the home. Their social role kept them focusing on the family and home with occasional charitable work for the church. (Uribe, 2008, pp. 27–28)

CONCLUSION

Completing a nursing history dissertation is possible with consideration for the special issues that arise. This chapter helps to explain some of the potential technical obstacles that need to be overcome and, I hope, can get you past issues that stand in your way. Much more remains to be analyzed about the profession of nursing, our leaders, and our responsibility in the health care system.

REFERENCES

Allende, S. (1939). *La realidad medico-social chilena: Síntesis* [The medico-social reality Chilean: Synthesis]. Santiago, Chile: Ministerio de Salubridad, Prevision, y Asistencia Social [Ministry of Health, Welfare and Social Assistance].

Barr-Melej, P. (2001). *Reforming Chile: Cultural politics, nationalism, and the rise of the middle class.* Chapel Hill, NC: University of North Carolina Press.

Clappison, G. (1964). *Vassar's Rainbow Division, 1918.* Lake Mills, IA: Graphic Publishing Company.

Collier, S., & Sater, W. F. (2001). *A history of Chile, 1808–1994.* Cambridge, UK: Cambridge University Press.

de Ramón, A. (2001). *Breve historia de Chile: Desde la Invasión Incaica hasta nuestros días* [Brief history of Chile: From the Inca invasion to the present day] *(1500–2000).* Buenos Aires, Argentina: Editorial Biblos.

Drake, P. (1973). The Chilean socialist party and coalition politics, 1932–1946. *The Hispanic American Historical Review, 53*(4), 619–643.

Dreves, K. D. (1975). Nurses in American history: Vassar training camp for nurses. *American Journal of Nursing, 75*(11), 2000–2002.

Flores, R. (1965). *Historia de la enfermería en Chile: Síntesis de su evolución educacional* [History of nursing in Chile: Synthesis of their educational development]. Santiago, Chile: I.a. Parte.

Frakia, E. (1943). El centro de salud y la enfermería [The health and nursing]. *Revista de Asistencia Social* [Journal of Social Assistance], *12*(1), 37–53.

Lanza Lazcano, C. (1998). *Breve Esbozo Histórico de la Enfermería en Chile* [Brief Historical Sketch of Nursing in Chile]. Unpublished manuscript, Centro de Documentación [Documentation Center], Colegio de Enfermeras de Chile [Colleges of Nurses of Chile]. Santiago, Chile.

Laval, E. (1944, Julio-Diciembre [July-December]). Don Alejandro del Río. *Revista de Asistencia Social* [Journal of Social Assistance], XIII, 135–270.

Ley 6174. (1938, Septiembre [September]). *Medicina Preventiva,* Artículo 1 y 2, Biblioteca del Congreso Nacional de Chile [Preventive Medicine, Article 1 and 2, Library of Congress of Chile].

Monteón, M. (1998). *Chile and the great depression: The politics of underdevelopment, 1927–1948.* Tempe, AZ: Arizona State University Press.

Paden, R. (1934, October 19). [Station Letter]. Presbyterian Historical Society (RG 160, Series 9, Box 4, Folder 25), Philadelphia, PA.

School for social workers: Maintained by Simmons College and Harvard University. (1905). *American Journal of Nursing, 5*(8), 512.

Uribe, J. (2008). *Nurses, philanthropies, and governments: The public mission of Chilean nursing, 1900–1945* (Doctoral dissertation). Retrieved from Proquest, UMI Dissertation Publishing. (3309517)

Wahatoya Huerfano County Yearbook. (1912). [Yearbook]. Retrieved from http://www.kmitch.com/Huerfano/yearbook1912/page 20.html

CHAPTER FIVE

CONDUCTING ORAL HISTORY RESEARCH IN COMMUNITY MENTAL HEALTH NURSING

Geertje Boschma

Iregularly use oral history in my research on the history of nursing and health care. It has proven to be a successful approach in making known the perspectives and experiences of people who most closely experienced social change (Thompson, 2000). These perspectives are often overlooked in traditional historiography, which can contribute to an incomplete understanding of health care history (Bornat, Perks, Thompson, & Walmsley, 2000). Understanding the development of community mental health care during the second half of the 20th century, for example, would be incomplete without the viewpoint and voice of consumers and frontline workers (Fingard & Rutherford, 2011; Tomes, 2006).[1] Oral history is thus both an empowering and innovative approach to writing a more inclusive account. As a platform from which to explore oral history methodologies, in this chapter I focus, in particular, on the role of community mental health nurses drawing on an oral history study I recently completed (Boschma, 2012). The perspectives of consumers and families have been included in other study reports (Boschma, 2013; Boschma, Haney, & Gorrie, 2012).

Parts of this chapter are drawn from Boschma, G. (2012). Community mental health nursing in Alberta, Canada: An oral history. *Nursing History Review*, 20: 103–135; and Boschma, G., Scaia, M., Bonifacio, N., & Roberts, E. (2008). Oral history research. In S. B. Lewenson & E. Krohn-Herrmann (Eds.), *Capturing nursing history: A guide to historical methods in research* (pp. 79–98). New York: Springer Publishing. I thank Mary de Chesnay, Sandra Lewenson, and reviewers for their generous comments on earlier drafts of this chapter.

Collecting people's personal stories by tape or video recorder gained momentum as a historical research approach in the 1970s when historians, coming from a critical social stand, began to explore the voices and stories of ordinary people often overlooked in traditional historiography (Grele, 2006; Perks & Thomson, 2006). It helped to understand social changes and events from a "bottom-up" rather than a "top-down" perspective (Grele, 2006; Kerr, 2003). Oral history has developed in close interdisciplinary relation with other fields in the humanities and social sciences, evolving in the interrelated approaches of oral history, life stories or life history, biography, and narrative analysis (Abrams, 2010; Boschma, Scaia, Bonifacio, & Roberts, 2008). Often oral history sources are complemented by existing written documentation and archival sources to obtain a rich collection of evidence about particular social developments and cultural and life events. Interviews provide a unique source of created evidence offering an interpretation of past events as co-constructed in the interview by interviewer and interviewee. The account is never a factual story of what happened but provides a recollection structured by memory, later events, present experiences and circumstances, and the relationship between researcher and interviewee; it must be analyzed as such for meaning. Oral history allows for examination of the way people have experienced past events and how they remember them requiring careful interpretation and reflection on the influences structuring the interviews (Portelli, 2006; Thomson, 2011). Relying on analytic frameworks from cultural and literary studies, oral history has grown into a socially critical and complex analytic practice (Chamberlain, 2006; Tonkin 1992). Oral history accounts assist researchers in gaining an intimate understanding of practical experiences and dilemmas from the perspective of people who experienced them.

In the study of community mental health nurses' experiences, for example, it helped me to learn that the nurses involved in community mental health settings actually had prior experience working in institutions. By means of the analysis of their account of their past experiences, I understood how these experiences influenced their perspective on the development of community-based services and how they felt services for patients or consumers in the community could best be developed. Furthermore, the interpretation of the interviews becomes richer and more meaningful if the researcher has a good understanding of the contextual literature and secondary historical sources of the time period and events under study. Such contextual knowledge not only shapes the interview questions and the discussion during the interview but also informs the questions raised during the analysis and interpretation.

DESCRIPTION OF THE STUDY

Summary of the Study

The study investigated how the emphasis in psychiatric care shifted from a trend toward the institutionalization of patients to a community service approach from the 1960s onward in one Canadian province. Oral history interviews were included to explore how community mental health nurses understood and created their new role and identity in the turbulent context of deinstitutionalization. These interviews complemented examination of written documents and other archival material. The development of so-called "after-care services" for patients discharged from Alberta Hospital Ponoka (AH-Ponoka), a large mental institution in the middle of the Canadian province of Alberta, to the city of Calgary in southern Alberta during the 1960s and 1970s formed the core focus. I specifically focused on the establishment of outpatient services in a new psychiatric department at the Foothills General Hospital in Calgary. Second, I examined how deinstitutionalization itself shaped community mental health nurses' work. On the basis of my analysis, I concluded that new rehabilitative, community-based mental health services can be better understood as a transformation of former institutional practices rather than as a definite break with them.

Conceptualizing the Study

Historical research, similar to other approaches, starts with a question that guides the investigation. In historical inquiry, the question informs the exploration of existing literature as well as decisions about the archival collections or other sources that might help answer the question. Part of this decision is also whether oral history should be included or whether oral history might perhaps be the primary focus. Sometimes little written evidence exists, and oral history seems the best approach to understand a particular change or event. The overarching question that guided my project in this particular case was: What are the important local, regional, national, and international influences that brought about change in psychiatric care and responses to mental illness? I focused on developments (and archives) in Alberta as a case study. I then asked further questions about the experiences of families and health care professionals, which, in this study, led me to explore specifically the experiences of community mental health nurses, a role that was newly developed in the transition from institutional to community-based care. Guided by a broader social history framework, I was particularly interested in how place and identity had shaped their experiences.

In the post-World War II era, mental health care policy shifted from large, remote institutions toward community-oriented services and general hospital psychiatry, most often centralized in urban areas. Still, deinstitutionalization increased reliance on psychiatric departments in general hospitals, and more community services have not resolved the complex problems people living with mental illness continue to face including stigma, homelessness, disparities in access, and lack of specialized services (Kirby, 2005). I argued how the shift to community settings had produced new, more fluid, but perhaps equally complex institutional contexts, questioning whether we really can speak of a process of deinstitutionalization. It seemed that the persistent dilemmas had been reproduced in the community. In this study my goal was to better understand this dilemma through the lens of the work of nurses. Place and identity were key concepts guiding the analysis (Elliott, 2004; Elliott, Stuart, & Toman, 2008). The study has been built upon a broad historiography examining the relationship between families, professionals, and institutions as a complex and dynamic interplay shaped by multiple social and cultural influences (Bartlett & Wright, 1999; Boschma, 2013; Grob, 1994; Moran, 2000; Moran & Wright, 2006). Careful listening to oral history accounts of frontline professionals and family members deepens our understanding of the development of mental health care (Boschma, 2007). Stories present an important framework for understanding the process of identity formation. We now have a rich body of contextual literature on oral history that provides guidance and context for the analysis and interpretation of the interviews (Boschma et al., 2008).

Because oral history is both a framework and a method, any oral history account needs careful analysis. It is not only an interview technique but also a particular approach to the interpretation of the narrative created from the interview. The analysis of oral history interviews closely aligns with approaches of textual analysis and narrative interpretation (Abrams, 2010; Mann Wall, 2006). The story of Margaret Mandryk in this study illustrated this point. The analysis of her story helped to understand and guide the analysis of the remainder of the interviews. A story is always a "construction" in which people express their identity and beliefs, and share what the experience meant to them. Opinions, emotions, and values about practices, experiences and approaches change over time as do practices themselves (Perks & Thomson, 2006; Thompson, 2000; Yow, 2005). Therefore, it is important to not only note *what* nurses said, but also *how, when, and in what context* in the interview. Mandryk, for example, participated in our oral history project with psychiatric mental health nurses in Alberta in the late 1990s.[2] We had a semistructured set of questions to guide the interview, starting with a question about the interviewee's early career and education in the mental hospital training school for psychiatric nursing. We were more focused on the context of the mental hospital rather than community mental health care. In response, Mandryk told us how she started her nursing career at Alberta Hospital in Edmonton in 1962 at age 18. Our question likely guided her to share her memories about her training school experience, which was fairly typical for nurses at the time. Mandryk shared how she was living in residence, thriving on friendships in a close-knit, relatively isolated community of fellow student nurses: "It was quite a feat to live in the country and take a bus trip into Edmonton ... I think there was one gal that had a car" (Mandryk, 1999). Turnover was high, she remembered, as the work environment was challenging, and many left:

> ...so you know, being eighteen and going into a mental institute where medications are not like what they are now, it sort of wakes you up very quickly to .... Well having these big, big groups of people, and I'm talking probably thirty people, ... on a ward and having people just sitting around and they certainly had some programs but a lot of the day was just spent sitting, and for the ... the age of patients, certainly a lot of older people ... and, um, when the young people came in for admissions and stuff ... how horrifying it must have been for them to sleep in a dormitory and have all of these people you know, sitting. (Mandryk, 1999)

Thinking about this time during the interview, more than 30 years later, Mandryk shared with us aspects of her work in the institution that in retrospect had come to be seen as the more negative, custodial aspects of institutional care. Although she was careful in pointing out how circumstances at the time shaped nurses' work, she might also have been thinking about what we likely expected to hear, considering how the common perspective on that time period in psychiatric history had changed. But then, almost out of the blue, Mandryk shifted the topic in the interview; in the middle of talking about the treatments at the time, the use of paraldehyde for sedation, insulin therapy, hydrotherapy, and unmodified shock therapy, she said: "... well, I graduated in 1965 and [moved to Calgary]," and started to talk about how she began working in mental health in Calgary, interrupting the flow of talk, perhaps to distance herself from a way of practice that, in retrospect, seemed limited to her. In interrupting the flow, she also pushed the interviewer to take into consideration a different perspective: Mandryk's career path was not only a story about institutional care, but also one about change toward community care. She wanted the interviewer to listen to the story that was important to her. She focused on her move to Calgary, almost as if shaking off a way of working she no longer identified with. As she took on a new position in Calgary, her identity changed. She powerfully evoked how she became Calgary's first community mental health nurse, a new identity she actively embraced in 1966, but likely also one that was not even described that way then. At that time, she was most likely called a psychiatric nurse. Only in retrospect did she use the phrase "community mental health nurse," as it was in retrospect that she related to a transforming identity, a shifting context, for which the seeds, however, were already planted in the third and last year of her training... : "even by my third year [in the mental hospital] things were a lot different in what we were studying, ... looking at more things like the social factors of life, things like alcoholism." They moved away from the straight focus on anatomy and medications of the first year, she remembered.

Another formative influence during her training was a taste of community work she had been able to get, as by the mid-1960s, the Alberta Hospitals both in Edmonton and Ponoka had begun to downsize and discharge their chronic mentally ill population:

> I did some community, a little bit of work with a social worker there at Alberta Hospital in Edmonton as part of my um, I think it was an elective, ... really enjoyed community work and often thought gee that would be what I [would like to] do when I graduate, but again, you just, you just sort of dream about those sort of things, and when I came to Calgary I started to look for work, there wasn't a whole lot open for psychiatric nurses. (Mandryk, 1999)

What she dreamed of was not readily available. Inspired by those experiences, however, Mandryk preferred to stay in psychiatry. Because Calgary did not have a large mental hospital, jobs for psychiatric nurses were not readily available. She persisted, perhaps aware of the fact that AH-Ponoka was actually discharging patients to Calgary, which was coordinated at the Guidance Clinic.[3] She explored her options: "I just phoned, started to phone places." She phoned the Guidance Clinic, where she got in touch with a social worker who asked her to come in and have an interview: "we hit it off so well that she phoned [the AH-Ponoka] and said look, I'm too busy, [...] She says

I'm too busy, I don't know medications, I don't know this, [...] I want you to hire Margaret Mandryk."

The social worker may indeed have had a keen interest in getting some help from a psychiatric nurse, who actually understood these clients and the medications they were on, which now needed monitoring, if not administering, in the community. Mandryk's experience was valued: "And so I went to AH-Ponoka, I think the next Tuesday ... we traveled to AH-Ponoka every Tuesday [to coordinate discharges] and we went to AH-Ponoka the next Tuesday and they hired me and that's how I had my job." A new era of community mental health nursing began for Mandryk. She would take on a key role in constructing and shaping it, as nurses trod new ground in a grassroots development of skill and service in the community. In her story, we can trace the larger social changes of which she was part. Her individual options were structured by the social, cultural, and institutional influences of the time.

ORAL HISTORY: METHODOLOGICAL FEATURES

Memory

An often raised question about oral history research is whether oral evidence drawn from memory can be trusted because of its subjective nature (Grele, 2006). Indeed, recalling past events and sharing memories is influenced by the present. The narrator and interviewer create historical evidence in a dynamic process of co-constructing. Current life events of the narrator as well as the environment in which the story is told may influence the story. Also, the nature of the relationship between the narrator and the researcher has an effect because it involves power dynamics. The relationship between interviewer and interviewee also influences the interpretation (Borland, 2006; Perks & Thomson, 2006; Sugiman, 2006). Oral historians have persuasively argued that oral and written sources are equally credible but different in nature (Charlton, Myers, & Sharpless, 2006; Radstone & Schwartz, 2010).

Joyce Taylor (pseudonym), one of the nurses in the study, illustrated the complex, yet essential, contribution of subjective memories to the understanding of the past very well. She shared her memories not because of her own experiences, but because of those of her clients (Taylor, 2004). She wanted to stay anonymous, but she chose to participate because she felt that otherwise the experiences of the people who had made the transition from institution to community—people, often at an older age, after having spent years, if not decades, in the institution—would not be heard. In her story she reconstructed leaving as a challenge. Her account also gives a unique insight into the meaning of self-help in community care.

Despite the optimism with which community care was developed, many of the former patients ended up quite isolated once again, and not all received the support they needed, Taylor explained. Her stories about her clients illustrated how the formerly hospitalized patients were still not well when they moved into the community, and they were not always able to get the support they needed. In the more unpredictable context of the community, support was a complex process not only to create or provide but also to get. Patients appeared visible only when they connected to a clinic or agency on a regular basis but there was no guarantee this would actually happen. Taylor followed patients who came to the Foothills General Hospital's psychiatric clinic in Calgary on a monthly or biweekly basis. The psychiatrist leading the follow-up program ran a group for schizophrenic patients. During their visit, the patients attended the group, saw the psychiatrist individually if necessary, and also saw the nurse. Taylor worked primarily with elderly individuals, who were in their seventies at the time of their discharge from AH-Ponoka: "they were becoming elderly because, you know, they'd been in AH-Ponoka for so many years, so we're looking at people in their seventies." Sometimes reinstitutionalization [in nursing home or lodge] occurred as these elderly clients became too frail. One frail older woman Taylor visited in the community on a regular basis "was somebody, you know, that survived, just barely survived; so when she became extremely frail, we were actually able to get in the geriatric mental health team, and they moved her to a nursing home to spend her last days." Taylor continued to point out that getting people with a psychiatric diagnosis into a nursing home was very difficult at the time, but also essential: "I was having to move a lot of these people into nursing homes because they just were not surviving on their own and there wasn't family support."

Taylor observed how people were functioning during home visits, and she tried to revitalize connections with siblings or sometimes with children of the discharged person. Occasionally, she was able to find families, but "they didn't understand, they weren't given the, the teaching about schizophrenia ... and so this particular [elderly] lady had a sister and a brother I was able to contact regarding her care, but you had to do a fair amount of pushing to get ... to get the family involved." Clearly guided by a holistic philosophy of care, she pointed out: "that's to illustrate that, you know ... there's a lot of total care that has to be done for people, you know, they may be able to live in the community sort of, but not ... not well" (Taylor, 2004).

The older woman who Taylor visited,

> ...was [living] in a very, very poor basement apartment, very drafty, you know, not good living conditions. She had never thought to let us know at clinic that there was a roommate there and the roommate was a lady who was more elderly than herself who had been in AH-Ponoka for years and years and years and the two of them were discharged around the same time and moved in together. [...] The roommate never got any treatment at all and became extremely paranoid [...] she had all her stuff in piles all over with signs everywhere do not touch, do not come near here. ... So when I went to visit and discovered this woman she was very unkempt and very suspicious of me. My patient had been trying to, you know, bring in food and look after her as they aged [...]. (Taylor, 2004)

A "self-help" philosophy sometimes emerged out of necessity, and peer help was a crucial survival strategy (Shimrat, 1997). Emerging patterns of self-help, which could also be framed as survival strategies, have been looked upon both in positive and negative terms and are at the heart of the consumer movement that grew in the context of deinstitutionalization (Tomes, 2006). For some, these developments underscored how psychiatry did not work, and that, as a result, consumers or survivors had to rely on each other, in a context where actual resources were lacking. Others saw self-help as the beginning of a more independent life in the community, provoking healthy coping mechanisms that helped people with mental illness to recover and survive (Knowles, 2000; Tomes, 2006).

This ambivalence is further illustrated in Taylor's story about one other client she worked with:

> ...who "was in a bachelor suite in a very run ... down apartment, he had one of these tiny little fridges, he only ate canned foods, ... His nutrition was a problem, he was getting older, he was in his seventies and financially wise, I mean there was money but the trustee had it ... sending him ... enough to pay for his rent and [...] food ... he would get some notices from the trustee that there was such and such an interest due but he had delusions about this money, he, he was ripping up any notices that he got from the trustee so, you know. ..." Only after careful negotiation with the trustee and the relatives, backing herself up with medical power, arguing how the doctor wanted better living conditions for the client, was Taylor able to get her client "some nice furniture and

a colored television and a remote and, you know, some nice things" and with some further effort, she got "him to move to another senior's apartment complex. (Taylor, 2004)

The stories of home visiting work illustrate a number of points. First, they show how the strategy to actively help people socialize, as well as the pressure former patients felt falling upon themselves to survive in a new context of "community," pushed a new agenda of rehabilitation, in which people with mental illness took on an active role in the management of their lives and care. Second, as both Taylor and Mandryk's stories showed, rehabilitation provided nurses the opportunity to construct a more independent, therapeutically based professional identity. Finally, the stories also illustrate how the ideal of independence in the community was fragile, difficult to achieve, and fraught with many new problems as the demand for community care increased and resources fell short. Many of the dilemmas and challenges of long-term institutional care were reproduced rather than resolved in the new community-based mental health services.

Sampling and Recruitment

Another decisive influence on any oral history project is the approach to recruitment and sampling of interviewees. Most oral historians use purposeful sampling to select participants. Participants are selected because of the representativeness and uniqueness of their experiences, not because of the generalizability of the findings. Individuals are included on the basis of personal knowledge of the event or phenomenon and their ability and willingness to communicate this experience to others (Abrams, 2010; Sandelowski, 1995). Therefore, networking and building relationships within the field are important aspects of purposeful sampling to find participants. In my study, I used word of mouth and purposeful sampling to recruit participants, with help from community partners. I gave brief presentations about the study at several community mental health agencies, and some of my colleagues also helped spread the word. I prepared a brief one-page announcement of the study to be distributed. This strategy also was useful from an ethical point of view; people were not directly approached by the researcher but by means of a third party. This was to avoid any undue pressure to participate, while giving people a chance to ask questions. People who did respond were clearly interested in sharing their stories and felt it was important to do so, which aligned with similar observations in the oral history literature: People who choose to participate generally do so because they want to share the story that is important to them (Portelli, 2006). Depending on the purpose of the interview, if an interview guide is developed, it typically has broad open questions so the interviewee can direct the course of the interview and actually tell the story that is important to him or her (Anderson & Jack, 2006). Furthermore, collecting some basic biographical information also is advisable.

Collecting Oral Histories and Consent

Consent is a key aspect of oral history research. Because of interviewees' participation in oral history research, ethical guidelines and regulations governing research involving human subjects have to be followed and informed consent must be obtained prior to the start of the interview process. Because participants are often selected because of their identity and experience, oral history interviews are usually not anonymous, and the information that the interviewee shares might not be confidential (Yow, 2005). Researchers have to develop an ethical protocol for their research that outlines how they will handle the confidentiality of the stories they collect. It is imperative that researchers consult with their local institutional ethics board and develop a protocol that not only meets the locally established ethical guidelines but also fits the purposes of the oral history project. Sometimes, it is important to protect the identity of the interviewee and provide the participants with the option to have their name revealed or stay anonymous. In this study some participants purposefully chose to not have their identity revealed. Nevertheless, their stories provide a valuable contribution to the history of the experience of living with mental illness from a family point of view. Using pseudonyms and excluding identifiable information from the accounts can be a valid and, sometimes, necessary oral history research strategy.

Consent in oral history has two aspects (Boschma, Yonge, & Mychajlunow, 2003; Shopes, 2006). First, the interviewee must be fully informed about the purpose and procedures of the oral history interview to consent to participate in the interview. Second, because most often the purpose of an oral history interview is to preserve the interview for future research and store the tapes and transcripts in a permanent repository, an existing archive, or digital collection, participants must be informed about how the information is used, and they must consent to preservation and release of the interview accordingly. For this particular study, the Behavioral Research Ethics Board of the University of British Columbia granted ethical approval. The consent provided participants the option of either having their name or a pseudonym used. I also gave people the option to have the interview used for this particular research only, for this research and my future research projects, or to have it additionally preserved for future research by depositing the interview in an archive upon completion of the study.

Preservation of Oral History

Preservation of nurses' stories can be an objective in and of itself, especially if nurses have work experiences in an area of health care that is rapidly changing. Often, certain areas of nursing work are more emphasized than others when the historical role of nursing in health care is highlighted. Nurses' work in mental health care has long been an understudied area in nursing history (Boschma, 2013). Oral history projects can help to highlight important transformations in psychiatric mental health or other areas of health care from the vantage point of nurses (Toman, 2001). Preserving stories of nurses who cared for mentally ill patients in either institutional settings or community services in Alberta between 1940 and 1990 was an explicit goal in a previous oral history project (Boschma, Yonge, & Mychajlunow, 2003). One of the first oral history projects with nurses was started by the Royal College of Nursing in the United Kingdom in the 1980s, followed by the more recent Nurses' Voices project (McCubbin & Warsop, 2010).

ANALYSIS AND INTERPRETATION OF ORAL HISTORY: WHOSE VIEWS?

Interpreting nurses' experience with mental health services and the way they participated in shaping them was at the heart of my project on the history of mental health care. In the process of interpretation, I relied heavily on narrative approaches (Abrams, 2010; Boschma, 2007; Chamberlain, 2006). The researcher examines the way cultural and social meaning is embedded in the stories and what the language conveys about the larger social structures and power relationships the individual is part of. Interpretation of oral history is not about imposing a preconceived framework upon the evidence but rather an effort to reveal the meaning embedded in the stories. Narrative interpretation seeks to understand how the subjective, individual experiences of ordinary people are both shaped by and are exemplars of larger social processes. The eventual interpretation offered in the published report is typically that of the researcher. In narrative analysis, Thompson (2000) notes, the interview is treated as a text and concerns itself with "language, its themes and repetitions, and its silences, [and] how the narrator experienced, remembered, and retold his or her life-story, and what light this may throw on the consciousness of the wider society" (p. 270). Narrative interpretation of personal accounts, whether from consumers, family members, or nurses, can foster a critical understanding of our collective consciousness and broader disciplinary discourses around important life experiences, such as dealing with mental illness, as well as the construction of disciplinary nursing knowledge and practice. The latter point was illustrated in the study, for example, in the way nurses conveyed their understanding of their role in monitoring and giving medication. Listening to (and interpreting) their stories, I understood this work as another driving force that structured nurses' understanding of their role and responsibility besides provision of rehabilitative support in the construction of "postasylum" community mental health nursing.

Larry Lyons, for example, a 1962 graduate from the mental hospital in Edmonton, Alberta, and the individual in charge of the admission ward, remembered: "I started outpatient care on the (mental hospital) unit and had our own staff follow-up the [discharged] patient. [...] On their way home. They would leave about an hour early or something like that. Go see the patient and give them an injection if they needed it or whatever was the case" (Lyons, 2000). As patients left the hospital, medication use was an important reason for psychiatric nurses to become involved in follow-up care because nursing or group home staff was unfamiliar with psychiatric patients. Lyons noted: "The [psychiatric nurses] would go down to the area that the patient was being considered for, talk with the staff ... alleviate any fears that the staff at the other [agency] might have." [Nurses] would help with the transitions of patients into the community and enjoyed that new responsibility: "We ... may go back into the community that way. It was growing. [...] [Nurses] were enjoying it. To them it was great and as a matter of fact today all of them are in community nursing now," Lyons emphasized. The excerpt reflects excitement about this new area of nursing work, which gave psychiatric nurses a more independent role in the community.

In the stories of the nurses involved in outpatient care at the Foothills General Hospital, another important point was that many patients who lived in the community came to the outpatient clinic in the general hospital for follow-up care and to receive their medication. This was particularly the case once injectable medication became available in the 1970s. Depot medication, injected once a week or bimonthly and releasing the active drug over the course of a week or 2 weeks, was a new phenomenon compared to the pills from the 1950s. Nurses built relationships with their patients, whether formerly discharged from AH-Ponoka or belonging to a new generation of patients who used general hospital psychiatric services from the onset of their illness, largely around their need to come into the clinic for weekly or biweekly injectable medication. Or nurses gave medication during home visits if patients could not come in. Ellen Madison (2008), a registered nurse working at the Foothills hospital, remembered:

> ...so I checked in on Monday and Friday [in the clinic] and [the other days] I was in the community the whole time and I gave injections out there and I assessed people in their daily living skills, how they were coping at home, um, some people suffered from depression, ... some [from] schizophrenia, ... I saw ... some of them weekly, others every four weeks it depended on their needs." During the home visit, Madison remembered, "we took a vial out, we had little kits, ... cosmetic bags and we had syringes in there and needles and swabs, alcohol swabs and band aids, also medications and then we had our Kardex with our orders on there and then I would go from house to house depending on the caseload. (Madison, 2008)

Patients were encouraged to come to the clinic at Foothills General Hospital for follow-up and to receive their medication, but not all were able, or willing to do so:

> ...the people that we gave injections to in the community were the ones that absolutely refused to come into the hospital; they were very, very sick and so we would take the medication to them, we tried to always encourage them to come into clinic, see the physician every time but that wasn't [always] possible because some people just refused to come or they were too ill, Madison remembered. (Madison, 2008)

Ray Farrell (2007), psychiatrist, and Doug Carnochan (2007), registered psychiatric nurse, both of whom had been involved with the Foothills hospital outpatient clinic from its infancy, called the coming of injectable medication "a major event."[4] They commented on the central role of injectable medication in structuring their patients' enduring connection to the clinic:

> ...still you saw the patient more frequently because you had to bring them in every week [...] to give them their shots. And that's much more frequently than people who ordinarily got followed up [...] and that was one of the most important aspects, I think, of the outpatient program system [...] as much as the medication itself, really [...]. (Farrell and Carnochan, 2007)

The pattern of taking pills 3 times a day, which had hitherto been the practice in community care, usually modeled after the general practitioner's practice of giving a prescription for 3 months, often made it challenging to maintain the connection with patients, they argued. Farrell remembered:

> ...our chief at the time, Dr. Pearce, um, [was] trying them as a novelty in these programs and, and being quite astounded at, [...] how few actual, uh, milligrams of the drug would do a person for a week compared with if you gave them pills three times a day. [The] actual load of medication that the patient got was vastly smaller and yet it was more effective. [...] you eliminated the element of, ... the person evading medication because of, uh, you know, because of their illness. [...] it was more compulsory in a way. (Farrell and Carnochan, 2007)

The administering of the depot dosage was more effective physiologically, and because it was more "compulsory," motivating patients to take pills three times a day was no longer needed. Nurses could now administer the necessary dosage in the clinic or during a home visit if need be. The institutional connection was a crucial element in making this technological system work.

Patients who needed injectable medication came in weekly or biweekly and allegedly developed a bond with the clinic. Carnochan commented: "[T]he frequency of visits was absolutely key in, in terms of having a person feel they belong to their own care." Nurses had to skillfully negotiate care and compulsion in such a way that it constructed the alleged community support patients needed. In the construction of community care, institutional practices had a powerful influence. For Farrell and Carnochan, the clinic served to recreate a sense of connection and belonging to a place that had meaning beyond the mere chemical substance of the medication. The injection bound the patient to an institutional context in a new, but perhaps also more fragile, way. As Farrell commented:

> ...the whole clinic system [was] part of a kind of a house of cards when one part ... leans to another and, and we do have a fairly elaborate system of approved homes, satellite homes, group homes, [...] merging into, ... almost nursing home type care. And, [...] those places would not be practical to run without our medication. And we couldn't run clinics without those places. ... Uh, they're kind of separate, but they are in[ter]dependent. (Farrell and Carnochan, 2007)

The metaphor of a house of cards in this quote seems significant. It suggests a reconstruction of an institutional context or system that sought to adapt to patient needs, largely relying on assumptions of support and supervision similar to that which underlay the traditional hospital but with a more fragile and fragmented nature. Outpatient clinics were complemented by inpatient services, which gradually obtained some of the traditional institutional features. As Farrell commented:

> ...the general hospital units in the 1960s made it a point of pride not to have any door that locked" ... "But gradually, more and more locks, more and more uh, shatterproof and, uh, special arrangements, uh, have made it so that [...] there's really no need to send anybody anywhere else on account of their violence of obstructiveness. (Farrell and Carnochan, 2007)

Farrell pointed out how general hospital psychiatry was not immune to the pressures brought about in dealing with the sometimes very difficult behaviors that accompanied mental illness. Whereas hitherto particularly difficult patients had been sent to AH-Ponoka when they could no longer be accommodated in the general hospital unit, gradually general hospital units themselves changed, incorporating some of the measures of force that had long characterized institutional psychiatric care.

Farrell's comment also illustrates the constraints and fragmentation under which the system of general hospital psychiatry and community care operated and developed, drawing a fine line between care and compulsion. Some of the dilemmas and challenges of long-term care were reproduced rather than resolved in the new community context of care. Although new services developed, along with more flexibility and community resources, more openness and education about mental illness, as well as better medication in some cases, the underlying physiology of mental illness remained largely unexplained, and the services did not evolve into a smooth, integrated system. The system provided nurses with new professional opportunities that excited them and allowed them to form a more independent professional identity in community mental health and general hospital clinics. But they also had to carefully negotiate how a sense of belonging and support for patients or clients could be constructed within the often limited and constrained parameters of postwar community mental health and general hospital psychiatry.

SUMMARY AND CONCLUSION

The stories of community mental health nurses, who had an essential role in developing new community services in Calgary, illustrated that new rehabilitative, community-based mental health services can be better understood as a transformation of former institutional practices rather than as a definite break with them. In the construction of these new services, nurses were able to carve out a new professional identity that expanded their independence, therapeutic role, and capacity for leadership. But the study also confirmed that establishing rehabilitation and community care in the 1960s and 1970s was a complex process constrained by pressures of funding and fragmentation (Fingard & Rutherford, 2011).

Oral history provides an important approach to gain an in-depth and contextual understanding of the way community mental health nurses understood and negotiated their new roles and responsibilities in the community. Careful interpretation of oral history interviews requires extensive submersion in the contextual historical literature, both in the historical context of the time period and the event under study and on the methodology (Nelson, 2002). Oral history has unique features of memory, consent, sampling, and preservation among other aspects. The example study well illustrated these elements. Analyzing the nurses' stories provided insight into the ways the larger processes of transition to community care constructed both the work of the nurses and the experiences of consumers. Ex-patients faced profound challenges once they had been transferred to a new community context. Institutional structures and inherent power dynamics did not disappear but resurfaced and were reproduced in new forms. Nurses' accounts of their experiences provide important insights into these dynamics and the larger transformation and restructuring of mental health care.

NOTES

1. I use the term *consumer* to refer to people living with mental illness. This is a more current term, reflecting the rise of the patient (or consumer) movement and one people with mental illness themselves currently use. For in-depth discussion of shifting terminology see Tomes (2006) and Fingard, and Rutherford (2011). Sometimes, I also use *patient* or *client* if that was the preferred terminology in an interview.
2. In the study on the work of community mental health nurses I included several interviews from a previous project designed to collect oral histories from psychiatric mental health nurses (Boschma, Yonge, & Mychajlunow, 2003). I augmented these with additional interviews conducted as part of this particular study.
3. Annual Report, Alberta Department of Public Health, Mental Health Division, 1966, p. 133. Provincial Archives of Alberta, Edmonton, Alberta.
4. Farrell had worked as a psychiatrist at the Foothills Department since 1967; Carnochan was a Registered Psychiatric Nurse. He graduated from AH-Ponoka in 1977, where he worked until 1978. That year he joined the staff at the Foothills Department, and had worked there since. It was their suggestion to be interviewed together.

REFERENCES

Abrams, L. (2010). *Oral history theory*. London, UK: Routledge.
Anderson, K., & Jack, D. C. (2006). Learning to listen: Interview techniques and analysis. In R. Perks & A. Thomson. (Eds.), *The oral history reader* (2nd ed., pp. 129–142). London, UK: Routledge.
Bartlett, P., & Wright, D. (1999). *Outside the wall of the asylum: The history of care in the community, 1750–2000*. London, UK: Athlone Press.
Borland, K. (2006). That's not what I said: Interpretive conflict in oral narrative research. In R. Perks & A. Thomson. (Eds.), *The oral history reader* (2nd ed., pp. 310–321). London, UK: Routledge.
Bornat, J., Perks, R., Thompson, P., & Walmsley, J. (Eds.). (2000). *Oral history, health and welfare*. London, UK: Routledge.
Boschma, G. (2007). Accommodation and resistance to the dominant cultural discourse on psychiatric mental health: Accounts of family members. *Nursing Inquiry, 14*(4), 266–278.
Boschma, G. (2012). Community mental health nursing in Alberta, Canada: An oral history. *Nursing History Review, 20*, 103–135.
Boschma, G. (2013). Community mental health post-1950: Reconsidering nurses' and consumers' identities. In P. D'Antonio, J. Fairman, & J. Whelan. (Eds.), *Routledge handbook on the global history of nursing* (pp. 237–258). London, UK: Routledge Taylor & Francis Group.
Boschma, G., Haney, C., & Gorrie, M. (2012). Gender, work and identity: Consumer perspectives on rehabilitation and recovery in mental health care. *The Bulletin of the UK Association for the History of Nursing, 1*(1), 9–20.
Boschma, G., Scaia, M., Bonifacio, N., & Roberts, E. (2008). Oral history research. In S. B. Lewenson & E. Krohn-Herrmann (Eds.), *Capturing nursing history: A guide to historical methods in research* (pp. 79–98). New York, NY: Springer Publishing.
Boschma, G., Yonge, O., & Mychajlunow, L. (2003). Consent in oral history interviews: Unique challenges. *Qualitative Health Research, 13*(1), 129–135.
Carnochan, D. (2007). Interview with Ray Farrell and Doug Carnochan by author, May 15, 2007.
Chamberlain, M. (2006). Narrative theory. In T. L. Charlton, L. E. Myers, & R. Sharpless (Eds.), *Handbook of oral history* (pp. 384–410). Lanham, MD: AltaMira Press.
Charlton, T. L., Myers, L. E., & Sharpless, R. (Eds.). (2006). *Handbook of oral history*. Lanham, MD: AltaMira Press.
Elliott, J. (2004). Blurring the boundaries of space: Shaping nursing lives at the red cross outposts in Ontario, 1922–1945. *Canadian Bulletin of Medical History, 21*(2), 303–325.
Elliott, J., Stuart, M., & Toman, C. (Eds.). (2008). *Place and practice in Canadian nursing history*. Vancouver, Canada: UBC Press.
Farrell, R. (2007). Interview with Ray Farrall and Doug Carnochan by author, May 15, 2007.
Fingard, J., & Rutherford, J. (2011). Deinstitutionalization and vocational rehabilitation for mental health consumers in Nova Scotia since the 1950s. *Histoire Sociale/Social History, 44*(88), 385–408.

Grele, R. J. (2006). Oral history as evidence. In T. L. Charlton, L. E. Myers, & R. Sharpless (Eds.), *Handbook of oral history* (pp. 43–101). Lanham, MD: AltaMira Press.

Grob, G. (1994). *The mad among us: A history of the care of America's mentally ill.* New York, NY: The Free Press.

Kerr, D. (2003). We know what the problem is: Using oral history to develop a collaborative analysis of homelessness from the bottom up. *Oral History Review, 30*(1), 27–45.

Kirby, M. J. L. (2005). Mental health reform for Canada in the 21st century: Getting there from here. *Canadian Public Policy: Analyse de Politique, 31*(s1), 5–12.

Knowles, C. (2000). *Bedlam on the streets.* London, UK: Routledge.

Lyons, L. (2000). Oral history interview with Larry Lyons, March 31, 2000, Alberta Association of Registered Nurses, Museum and Archives, Oral History Collection With Psychiatric Mental Health Nurses.

Madison, E. (2008). Interview with Ellen Madison by author, Calgary, February 25, 2008.

Mandryk, M. (1999). Oral history interview with Margaret Mandryk, September 7, 1999. Alberta Association of Registered Nurses, Museum and Archives, Oral History Collection With Psychiatric Mental Health Nurses.

Mann Wall, B. (2006). Textual analysis as a method for historians of nursing. *Nursing History Review, 14,* 227–242.

McCubbin, C., & Warsop, I. (2010). In K. Start, C. Quinn, & G. Aronin (Eds.), *Nurses' voices: Memories of nursing at St. George's hospital, London, 1930–1990.* London, UK: Faculty of Health and Social Care Sciences—Kingston University and St George's, University of London.

Moran, J. E. (2000). *Committed to the state asylum: Insanity and society in nineteenth-century Quebec and Ontario.* Montreal and Kingston, Canada: McGill-Queen's University Press.

Moran, J. E., & Wright, D. (Eds.). (2006). *Mental health and Canadian society: Historical perspectives.* Montreal and Kingston, Canada: McGill-Queen's University Press.

Nelson, S. (2002). The fork in the road: Nursing history versus the history of nursing. *Nursing History Review, 10,* 175–188.

Perks, R., & Thomson, A. (Eds.). (2006). *The oral history reader* (2nd ed.). London, UK: Routledge.

Portelli, A. (2006). What makes oral history different. In R. Perks & A. Thomson (Eds.), *The oral history reader* (2nd ed., pp. 32–42). London, UK: Routledge.

Radstone, S., & Schwartz, B. (2010). *Memory: Histories, theories, debates.* New York, NY: Fordham University Press.

Sandelowski, M. (1995). Focus on qualitative methods: Sample size in qualitative research. *Research in Nursing & Health, 18,*179–183.

Shimrat, I. (1997). *Call me crazy: Stories from the mad movement.* Vancouver, Canada: Press Gang Publishers.

Shopes, L. (2006). Legal and ethical issues in oral history. In T. L. Charlton, L. E. Myers, & R. Sharpless (Eds.), *Handbook of oral history* (pp. 135–169). Lanham, MD: AltaMira Press.

Sugiman, P. (2006). These feelings that fill my heart: Japanese Canadian women's memories of internment. *Oral History, 34*(2), 69–84, especially p. 71 and 82.

Taylor, J. (2004). Interview with Joyce Taylor (pseudonym) by Annette Lane, September 2, 2004. This interviewee preferred to be named by pseudonym.
Thompson, P. (2000). *The voice of the past: Oral history* (3rd ed.). Oxford, UK: Oxford University Press.
Thomson, A. (2011). Moving stories, women's lives: Sharing authority in oral history. *Oral History, 39*(2), 73–82.
Toman, C. (2001). Blood work: Canadian nursing and blood transfusion, 1942–1990. *Nursing History Review, 9*, 51–78.
Tomes, N. (2006). The patient as a policy factor: A historical case study of the consumer/survivor movement in mental health. *Health Affairs, 25*(3), 720–729.
Tonkin, E. (1992). *Narrating our pasts: The social construction of oral history.* Cambridge, UK: Cambridge University Press.
Yow, V. R. (2005). *Recording oral history: A guide for the humanities and social sciences.* Walnut Creek, CA: AltaMira Press.

Chapter Six

Celluloid Angels: The Power of Stories

David Stanley

The primary aim of this chapter is to discuss approaches to qualitative data analysis. Any qualitative study—ethnography, life history, grounded theory, phenomenology, historical research, participatory action research, or other qualitative approach to research—rests, to a large extent, upon the quality of the analysis that is applied to the data collected. Therefore, my primary aim is to guide the reader toward an appreciation of the often subtle but vital steps involved in qualitative data analysis. As part of this aim, I offer a description of the study—"Celluloid Angels: A Research Study of Nurses in Feature Films 1900–2007" (Stanley, 2008)—at the heart of this chapter. I discuss why and how the study outlined in "Celluloid Angels" was developed along with the challenges and issues faced in undertaking the study, and I offer the reader insight into how the challenges were overcome and how the qualitative aspects of the study were analyzed.

A GOOD STORY: HERODOTUS AND THE PHOENICIANS

Before I discuss my own research, I would like to start with a short story, for stories are at the heart of excellent qualitative research and they are indeed powerful. The following story is not mine. It was told in the most excellent and ancient of texts, *The Histories* by Herodotus. The introduction to *The Histories* begins:

> Herodotus' *Histories* is one of the most important works of Greek literature. Its importance lies not so much in its main subject, the battles fought by a number of Greek city states against an invading Persian army, as in the many stories drawn from Greek and non-Greek sources that Herodotus relates. (Herodotus, 1998, p. ix)

I would like to relate one of Herodotus's stories here. Herodotus narrates a story about the circumnavigation of Africa (when Herodotus wrote, Africa was known as "Libya"). He describes that it was known that Libya is washed on all sides by sea apart from where it is attached to Asia (very true) and that this was discovered by an Egyptian king called Necos, who sent a number of Phoenicians in ships east into the Arabian Sea with orders to make for the Pillars of Heracles (the entrance to the Mediterranean) by circumnavigating Africa and returning to Egypt. They were reported to have taken 3 years, stopping along the way to sow and gather crops when they went ashore. Herodotus then reports (although he declares that for his part he does not believe the Phoenicians) that in sailing around Libya they had the sun upon their right hand. Herodotus here shows himself as a faithful storyteller, for although he does not believe the story the Phoenicians tell, he faithfully retells it, unwittingly offering the evidence required for the story to be acknowledged as true. What the Phoenicians had done was sail far south of the equator to round Africa, and in the course of their journey the shadows from their sails were cast to the south of their ships—something that would be impossible if, as Herodotus (and most of the people living at this time) thought, the Earth was flat. The Phoenicians had not discovered that the Earth was round, but in their story, faithfully told by a doubting Herodotus, there was a gem of information that pointed to a new way to understand the world and perhaps even the place of the Earth within the universe.

This small example offers evidence of the power of stories. Qualitative data resonates with the power of stories. Many are personal, some are moving, and many simply tell one person's truth and knowledge about significant issues in their lives. However, the key to unlocking these stories is effective, detailed qualitative data analysis. Herodotus was a wonderful and faithful recorder of stories, but in his declaration that he did not believe the Phoenicians, he was abandoning analysis, and the people of the Mediterranean seeing the sun rise and fall to their south were to live for centuries more, believing the Earth to be flat. However, Herodotus was not a researcher. He was a storyteller and historian, and if qualitative researchers are to be seen as more than faithful storytellers, they need to develop and refine the art of analysis. For it is this aspect of qualitative research that changes a good story, a meaningful life event, or what could be quality data into valuable results and useful insights.

WHY LOOK AT FILMS? MY STORY

I have always loved movies and films. My formative years paralleled the development of TV and the explosion of the film and movie industry in the 1970s and 1980s. Now of course anyone can make a movie on his or her

CHAPTER 6. CELLULOID ANGELS: THE POWER OF STORIES   107

iPhone or with a GoPro camera or any digital camera and post it to YouTube via the Internet—never has the ability to tell a story via the visual media been greater. However, what do these visual stories tell us? As a male nurse I watched the films *Meet the Parents* and *Meet the Fockers* in the early 2000s with a mixture of respect for the acting, humor, and storyline of the films, and consternation at the message the films were sending about the role of men in nursing and how they seemed to support and promote negative stereotypes developed over the years about male nurses. As a male nurse, I found parts of the film were very difficult to watch, and I wondered if young men watching the films would be put off from considering nursing as a career. I wondered too what other films were saying or had said about nursing as a profession over the years. I could think of a handful of films that featured nurses or had nurses as a dominant part of their plot or story line, and thinking about the "Focker" films (a third film appeared in 2010 called *Little Fockers*), I was prompted to wonder about how nurses and nursing had been portrayed in feature films.

My initial interest in researching this topic began in late 2006, and in parallel with my own interest of how nurses were portrayed in films, I was required to develop a lecture for neophyte nursing students about how nurses were conceptualized by the nursing profession, other professions, and the public. I began by exploring existing literature about the topic, and found a number of nurse academics had also considered how the image of nurses was portrayed in the media (Bayer, 2007; Burech & Gordon, 2000; Farella, 2001; Ward, Styles, & Bosco, 2003). I read and searched widely for research focused papers and found a number of "opinion" papers that, while interesting, lacked research rigor, with only papers by Kalisch and Kalisch (1982), Kalisch, Kalisch, and McHugh (1982), and Darbyshire and Gordon (2005) offering detailed evidence of rigorous research studies of nurse-related feature films and their influence on the image of nurses and nursing. Feeling more was required, I began to design my own study.

STUDY DESIGN

The aim of the study was to explore how nursing and nurses were portrayed in feature films made between 1900 and 2007, with a nurse as their main or principal character and/or a story line related specifically to nursing. As such, the study had three objectives: first, to identify all feature films made between 1900 and 2007 that featured nurses or nursing as a main theme; second, to identify where each nurse-related film was produced, its genre, and its plot(s); and third, to identify the key themes from each of the films and explore how the image of nursing/nurses was being portrayed.

The various objectives of the research dictated that a mixed methodological approach be used. Quantitative analysis was employed to identify aspects of the research related to the number of films, country of production, genre, plot line, and other numerically obtainable data. However, to explore the themes related to how the image of nurses/nursing had been portrayed, a qualitative analysis using theoretical sampling (Strauss & Corbin, 1998) needed to be used.

In describing the research process, I often favor the use of figures or diagrams that outline the steps or phases of the research process, and in the "Celluloid Angels" article, the research process was set out visually. Figures allow the reader a quick visual reference of the research process and often provide a simplified snapshot of the whole study. Figure 6.1 is a simplified version of the diagram offered in the original article.

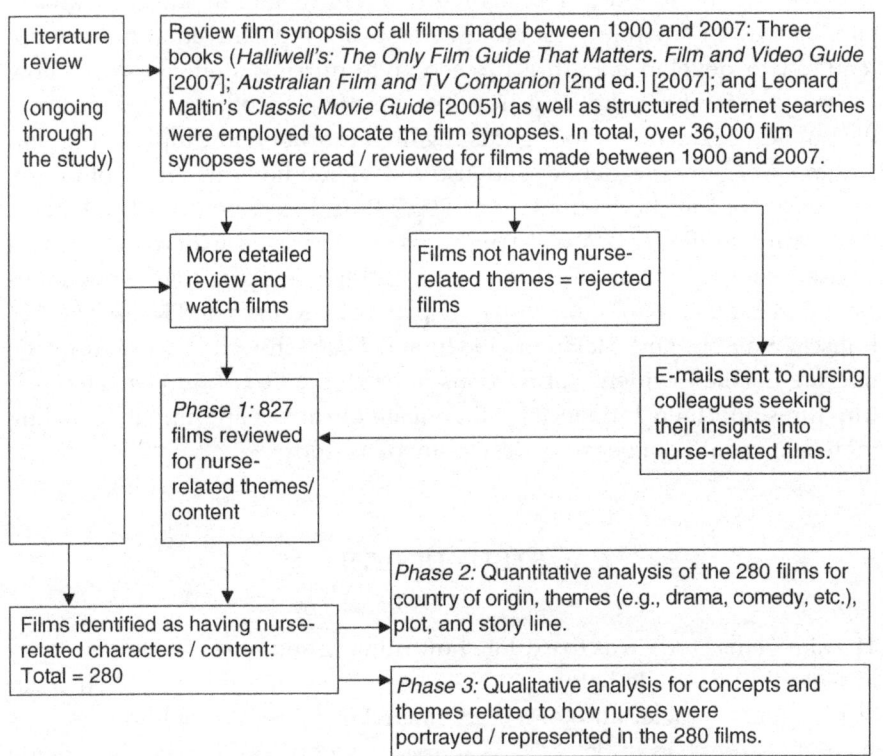

Figure 6.1 *A modified representation of the research process.*

QUALITATIVE DATA ANALYSIS: THEMES RELATED TO HOW THE IMAGE OF NURSES/NURSING WAS PORTRAYED IN FEATURE FILMS (1900–2007)

This paper deals only with the qualitative analysis in phase 3 of the study; however, this does not diminish the relationship between the qualitative and quantitative aspects of the mixed methods study as each is very much interdependent. As such, the qualitative phase of the study began after the quantitative data had been gathered and analyzed and started by regarding each film as a separate set of data (as if each were an individual interview or individual case). The first step of my qualitative data analysis was to watch or review each of the 280 films in detail (in the same way a qualitative researcher might read and review each interview transcript). Some films were not accessible, and so were reviewed via the Internet or via reviews about the films; however, the vast majority of films were watched and in some cases rewatched. Notes were taken about each film to help build a complete picture of the film's content, issues addressed, characterizations of the nurse or nursing roles, and concepts describing how nurses or nursing were portrayed. Initially, 34 concepts were identified, but this list was refined and shortened to 28 concepts after reevaluating each film and following consultation with a research partner, who independently reviewed the majority of the films. Needless to say, this process took many months, and apart from the task of actually reading each of the film synopses, this was by far the most laborious of the processes involved in the research. While initially frustrating, it was important that time was taken at this point to ensure that all the possible and potential concepts were captured and identified. The final 28 concepts identified are offered in Table 6.1.

Table 6.1 *Concepts Identified*

War nurse	Heroine	Self-sacrifice	Sex kitten
Call to duty	Object of desire	Romance	Unbalanced nurse
Nursing student	Novice nurse	Zombie nurse	Murdering nurse
Detective nurse	Missionary	Nun	Doctor/nurse relationship
Murder/Mystery	Sex object	Temptress	Strong woman
Nobody's fool	Children's nurse	Private nurse	Wit
Male nurse	Humor	Mothering nurse	
Specialist nurse (e.g., community/mental health/pediatrics)			

These concepts (or categories) were then explored for patterns or themes that pointed to how nurses had been portrayed on screen. The list of concepts was used as a guide to help group the concepts into themes. This task was again undertaken with the aid of an independent research assistant who confirmed the themes eventually identified. Eight themes were recorded: "self-sacrifice/care," "the heroine," "sex object," "romantic/feminine," "intelligent," "strong woman," "the dark nurse," and "the victim."

Many qualitative researchers use the term "emerged" at this point, as in, "the themes emerged from the data." Indeed, I used this term myself to describe the development of the themes in this study, and it is commonly used in research text describing qualitative data analysis, although I am not sure this term does justice to the effort the researcher needs to put into finding the concepts and then linking and building the themes. The data is clearly there awaiting exploration and extraction, labeling and identification, whereas the term "emerged" implies an almost magical or mystical process, like a rabbit being pulled out of a hat. This may be how the final themes appear, but the reality is that they only "emerge" after masses of careful consideration, hours and hours of sifting and sorting, and the most rigorous and detailed analysis. The real power of the stories that lie at the heart of qualitative data rests in the researchers' capacity to find their truth through the diligent and careful application of an appropriate analytical tool.

In analyzing the data for the "Celluloid Angels" study, I employed theoretical sampling (Strauss & Corbin, 1998). This approach is more commonly used in grounded theory studies (an area of qualitative research I have some experience in; Stanley, 2005, 2006), although this approach is being used more and more to gather and analyze data beyond grounded theory (Schneider, Whitehead, LoBiondo-Wood, & Haber, 2013). Polit and Beck (2012) describe theoretical sampling as a complex sampling technique that requires researchers to be involved in multiple lines and directions as they go back and forth between data and concepts (or categories) as the themes and potential theories emerge. They add that the purpose of data analysis is to arrange, structure, and elicit meaning from the data (Polit & Beck, 2012), and in many cases the task of analyzing the data can begin the moment the data collection begins, as it did with the "Celluloid Angels" study. There are many other frameworks and analytical approaches used in qualitative data analysis, with a number of researchers distinguishing between the analytical methods based upon their aims or focus. As such, some claim that conversational analysis, discourse analysis, symbolic interactionism, and ethnomethodology analytical tools focus on the use and interpretation of language. Others have adopted an interpretive analytical approach, which aims to understand and report on views and culture. Some researchers employ theory building approaches, such as grounded theory, in their analyses (Ritchie & Lewis, 2003). However, as Polit and Beck (2012, p. 557) note, regardless of the analytical approach or framework employed, "the analysis of qualitative data is an active and interactive process" requiring qualitative researchers to become completely familiar with and to carefully scrutinize and deliberately review their data in a search for understanding and meaning.

In the "Celluloid Angels" article, I made a point of including a table that linked the concepts and themes and added detail about the trend of themes over the years, as various themes seemed to be more or less dominant in various decades. The table (reproduced as a modified Figure 6.2) was important to include because it offers the reader a visual representation of the process of analysis, rather than simply offering a statement about the themes and hoping the reader will make the same leap I had made in identifying them.

Themes also appeared to vary in intensity, with a number of themes (e.g., "self-sacrifice/care," "the heroine," "sex object," and "romantic/feminine") appearing more commonly and consistently across the decades than the other themes identified (see Figure 6.2).

DESCRIPTION OF THE STUDY RESULTS: THE IMAGE OF NURSES/NURSING IN FEATURE FILMS

Films featuring nurses or nursing as a significant part of the film were identified in significant numbers, with 280 films being identified for inclusion in the study. The films offered up a wide range of plot and story lines, and nurses were shown or portrayed in a number of ways, often in either stereotypical and, in some, uncomplimentary roles, with these findings being supported with results from previous studies of a similar nature (Bayer, 2007; Burech & Gordon, 2000; Farella, 2001; Gordon & Johnson, 2004; Kalisch & Kalisch, 1982; Kalisch, Kalisch, & McHugh, 1982; Rasmussen, 2001).

Films from the early years of the 20th century portrayed nurses predominantly as heroines in romantic roles or as self-sacrificial carers, with World War I commonly used as a backdrop for the stories being told. These included films such as *Romance of a War Nurse* (1908), *The Woman the Germans Shot* (1918), *Dawn* (1928), *War Nurse* (1930), and *Nurse Edith Cavell* (1939). Nurses were also used for comedy or slapstick "chase" films that commonly portrayed nurses as sex objects (e.g., *Billy's Nurse* [1912] and *Why Worry?* [1923]), a theme that remained evident across the years. The themes of

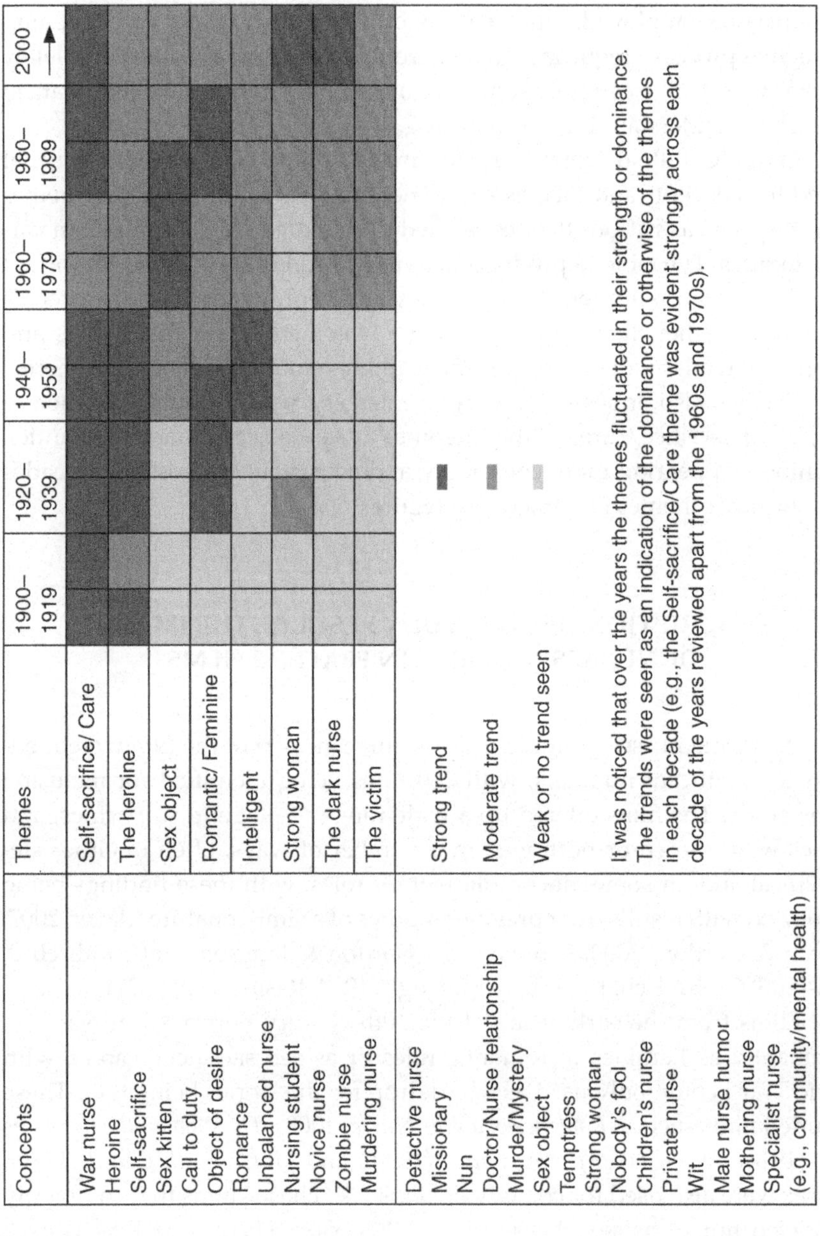

112   Nursing Research Using Historical Methods

Concepts	Themes	1900–1919	1920–1939	1940–1959	1960–1979	1980–1999	2000→
War nurse	Self-sacrifice/Care						
Heroine	The heroine						
Self-sacrifice	Sex object						
Sex kitten	Romantic/Feminine						
Call to duty	Intelligent						
Object of desire	Strong woman						
Romance	The dark nurse						
Unbalanced nurse	The victim						
Nursing student							
Novice nurse							
Zombie nurse							
Murdering nurse							
Detective nurse	Strong trend						
Missionary							
Nun	Moderate trend						
Doctor/Nurse relationship							
Murder/Mystery	Weak or no trend seen						
Sex object							
Temptress							
Strong woman							
Nobody's fool							
Children's nurse							
Private nurse							
Wit							
Male nurse humor							
Mothering nurse							
Specialist nurse (e.g., community/mental health)							

It was noticed that over the years the themes fluctuated in their strength or dominance. The trends were seen as an indication of the dominance or otherwise of the themes in each decade (e.g., the Self-sacrifice/Care theme was evident strongly across each decade of the years reviewed apart from the 1960s and 1970s).

Figure 6.2 *Concepts, themes, and trends over time.*

"self-sacrifice/care" and "the heroine" rarely faded from the crop of films reviewed, and apart from a lull in the 1960s and 1970s, these themes dominated many of the films studied throughout the century, reinforcing the nurse's core duty of being there for others. Also implied was the idea that as long as women (nurses) were kind, feminine, gave of themselves, and were nice, they had all that was required to be a nurse.

The other major theme seen throughout the century, but more prominently from the 1950s on, was that of "sex object." Kalisch and colleagues (1982) also indicated that this was a dominant theme of films about or featuring nurses, although some films were clearly more sexually provocative than others and, in some, humor and sexual flirtation could be seen to overlap. The implication of such a strong theme is that nursing as a profession and nurses in general are significantly tarnished by the proliferation of films showing nurses as objects of sexual desire. Films such as *Operation Petticoat* (1959), *Carry on Nurse* (1959), *The Hot Box* (1971), *Carry on Matron* (1972), *Rosie Dixon: Night Nurse* (1978), *Where the Money Is* (2000), *Yes Nurse, No Nurse* (2002), *Catch Me if You Can* (2002), and *Graveyard Alive: A Zombie Nurse in Love* (2005) continue to have an influence on how the nursing profession is perceived, with a potentially negative impact on perceptions of nurses' clinical practice and with a potentially unhelpful impact on nursing's aspirations to be taken seriously as a profession (Rasmussen, 2001).

However, it was noted that themes portraying nurses in feature films are moving away from the strong stereotypical themes of "the heroine," "self-sacrificial carer," and "sex object." In keeping with the evolution of the nursing profession, newer films are increasingly showing nurses to be empowered, professional, capable, intelligent, and strong, with films such as *The World According to Garp* (1982), *Magnolia* (1999), *14 Hours* (2004), and *Angels in America* (2005) demonstrating a move toward a more professional and competent portrayal of nursing.

Another, although thankfully minor, theme was that of "the dark nurse." This theme was seen in a range of films that show the more sinister side of nurses and nursing. The self-sacrificial and caring nurse theme remained more dominant, but it was noted that this was paralleled by a number of films that showed nurses as powerful, but evil, with some films being described as based on "real life events." A number of films demonstrating this theme seemed to be challenging the caring role of nurses or perhaps using this paradox to heighten the terror many of these films sought to offer. Examples of films demonstrating "the dark nurse" themes were *Woman of Straw* (1964). *The Honeymoon Killers* (1969), *Misery* (1991), *Blood: The Last Vampire* (2000), *Talk to Her* (2003), and *Silent Hill* (2007).

Films in the later years of the 20th century began to show a much wider range of characterizations of nurses and, to a large extent, mirror the changes evident in western society. Nurses in many films began to be seen beyond the self-sacrificial/care, sex object, heroine, and romantic roles and were increasingly seen as professionally competent, intelligent, witty, nobody's fool, or strong. Films such as *The World According to Garp* (1982), *Why Me?* (1984), *Intimate Strangers* (1986), *The English Patient* (1996), and the earlier scenes in *Talk to Her* (2002) offer examples of these changes in theme.

Also, nurse-related films in more recent years can be found with male nurses playing the nurse's role. Prior to the late 1960s I could locate no films with male nurses in them, and I located only seven films with men during this research. However, intrigued by this topic, I undertook a follow-up study, "Celluloid Devils: A Research Study of Male Nurses in Feature Films" (Stanley, 2012). In this more detailed study spanning films made up to 2011, I was able to locate 13 films that featured male nurses that, apart from one film (*Precious*, 2009), reinforced negative stereotypes and offered very disparaging images of men in the nursing profession. The aim of the follow-up study was to explore how men in nursing and male nurses were portrayed in feature films made between 1900 and 2011, with a male nurse as their main or principal character and a story line related specifically to men in nursing. Like the initial study, this also had three objectives: first, to identify all feature films made between 1900 and 2011 that featured a male nurse; second, to identify where each male nurse-related film was produced, its genre, and its plot(s); and third, to identify the key themes from each of the films and explore how the image of men in nursing and male nurses were being portrayed. I employed a similar methodological approach but also employed an interpretive approach guided by the framework of hegemonic masculinity. Given that only 13 films were located, a case study approach was overtly used to examine the portrayal of male nurses in feature films. I mention the follow-up study because it is an example of another qualitative study addressing a very similar topic to the "Celluloid Angel" study, but it employed a slightly different analytical approach reinforcing Polit and Beck's (2012) observation that the analysis of qualitative data is an interactive process requiring detailed scrutiny and with no universal rules.

The results of the qualitative analysis from the "Celluloid Angels" study indicated that, while the film image of nurses still resonates with nurses who are self-sacrificial, caring, romanticized, and seen as sex objects, more recent films offer a much wider range of characterizations with the role and image of nurses being expanded to accommodate nurses who are professionally sound, intelligent, strong, male, and with an overall more authentic representation of modern nurses and nursing being evident.

CHALLENGES AND ISSUES

Undertaking the research for "Celluloid Angels" presented a number of challenges and issues. The first related to the scope of the data identified. Usually in qualitative studies, interviews, focus groups, historical records, recorded information, and observations are the main sources of data. This type of data can yield masses of text and the "Celluloid Angels" data was no different. Although I had the advantage of not having to undertake copious interview transcriptions, the scope of the films' data, notes, and additional documents meant I was dealing with hundreds and hundreds of pieces of data. One of my first challenges was to manage a large quantity of data and arrange it so that I could interrogate it and reinterrogate the data appropriately and accurately. Simply put, my first challenge, as Polit and Beck (2012, p. 556) identified, was that qualitative analysis is "an enormous amount of work." As the study progressed, I realized that I had a mass of data to go through, and my commitment to complete the study was significantly challenged by the sheer amount of work involved.

I resolved this challenge by carefully labeling all of my work and dealing with each decade of film data separately. My home office was taken over by papers and notes about each film, all sorted into year-related piles. I also kept a corresponding set of computer files and similar notes that meant I could locate the information I needed by searching data for a specific 10-year period, rather than trying to locate data within the mass of notes and files all together. Later, once the themes were established, I broke the year-related data into smaller theme-specific sets of information, again helping with the process of managing all the data. My other strategy for dealing with all the data was to keep it at arm's length and not let it intrude on my life or overwhelm me. I took a very workmanlike approach to the data analysis, setting up a plan and sticking with it and working through each "decade" of data at a steady and regular pace without letting it get on top of me.

A significant issue for this study was that I was unable to locate and watch every one of the 280 films I had identified. Some were simply too old, and I did not have access to a vast film library, and others were simply rare films that I found difficult to locate. I overcame this drawback by accessing information online about the few films I could not watch or by watching excerpts of the films, again online. On a few occasions, the documentary information I was able to locate was also of poor quality, and while I tried to gather detailed information about every film, information about a few films remained scant.

There was no real solution to the problem of not being able to locate the films. I applied for a number of grants in the hope of being able to travel to larger film libraries but failed to secure the funds. In the end, all I could do was my best with the information I could locate. The Internet proved a reliable source of backup data and, fortunately, only a few films eluded me. The other step I took was acknowledging this as a limitation of the study in the original publication.

Another issue, common to qualitative data analysis, rests upon the language used to describe the categories and themes. For example, I used the term "sex object" as a concept or categorical descriptor when describing nurses who were seen in a sexually provocative or sexually alluring way in feature films. However, it could be that the language or words I used would not be the same as those that another researcher or someone else would have chosen to describe this observation; indeed, even the observation itself might not be viewed in the same way. This is particularly relevant as different cultures may have slightly different interpretations of some words or events, and this can change the meaning taken from the data analysis or the reading of the results. Numbers, used in quantitative data, are universally understood in any language although, as Polit and Beck (2012) indicate, no universal rules apply for qualitative data analysis.

A key to addressing this issue was to use aspects of the language used by previous researchers. Kalisch, Kalisch, and McHugh (1982) had used the term "sex object" in their research, and to be able to apply some consistency between their study and mine, I chose to use the same term. However, there are no rules, and researchers and writers will continue to apply their own terminology and cultural inflections as they describe their findings.

The final challenge, common to all qualitative data analysis, is that of reducing the data down to manageable and meaningful information so that the reader can understand and grasp the conclusions made as well as the process employed to reach those conclusions. The solution to this challenge is to be concise and accurate without losing the detail and richness of the data. The cost of not doing this is that often assumptions can be made about the process of data analysis. It is for this reason that documenting and laboring over an explanation of the analytical process is so vital in describing qualitative research. In a quantitative study, it may be appropriate to simply indicate that a T-test (e.g.) was applied in the analysis for the reader to grasp the significance of the results. Although this is rarely the case with qualitative data, it is incumbent upon the researcher to describe not just the results but the process of analysis that led to the "emergence" of the results, as I tried to do.

In general, most of these challenges and issues were overcome with the application of rigor, diligence, and hard work, and with the use of a clear analytical process as described in Figure 6.1.

PERSONAL REFLECTION

The study described here started life innocuously enough. It was not part of a PhD or masters project and it was not funded by any external or professional body. I saw a few films that got me thinking about how others might see nursing and how these films might influence people's perceptions of nurses or nursing, and then serendipity played a hand when I was asked to develop a lecture related to the very issues I had been contemplating. These issues tapped into a long-standing personal fascination with films and movies, and once I had *Halliwell's: The Only Film Guide That Matters* (Walker, 2006) in my hand, I was hooked and found myself on my own circumnavigation of films about nurses/nursing and then, in the second study, about films related to men in nursing. I had no idea what lay ahead, what stories I might find, or what the data would offer up. I just knew I wanted to go on this journey of discovery. I guess this is the first and most important step for any researcher, whether his or her focus is in the quantitative, qualitative, or mixed methods domain. The first key is to have an interest in or be passionate about discovery, because research, qualitative or quantitative, is focused on achieving the same ends: discovering or revealing the truth. The second key is that this can only be achieved by analysis of the facts or details of the data in a way that demonstrates rigor, trustworthiness, attention to truth telling, and long hours of honest sifting, sorting, and categorizing data.

CONCLUSION

My aim with this chapter was to solidify in the reader's mind the vital importance of analyzing qualitative data. Quantitative data often stands alone or unchallenged with the truth of the data being self-evident in the figures, numbers, tables, and graphs that commonly accompany quantitative studies. It is for this reason that quantitative data is often held aloft as the "gold standard" in the research pantheon. To gain credibility and lift the results from qualitative studies to equal heights, qualitative researchers need to reassert the power of people's stories that have been thoroughly and completely analyzed. The key to this is establishing a rigorous approach to data analysis (whichever framework or method of analysis the researcher uses) and then to lead the reader through the process of analysis so that the researcher's conclusions and analysis become equally self-evident to the reader. In the study outlined in this chapter, "Celluloid Angels: A Research Study of Nurses in Feature Films 1900–2007" (Stanley, 2008) and the follow-up publication, "Celluloid Devils: A Research Study of Male Nurses in Feature Films" (Stanley, 2012), I made every effort to not only analyze that data with care and rigor but to lead the reader through the steps I had taken in drawing my study conclusions. These are not always possible in every publication, but should be the aim of all qualitative researchers regardless. Both articles considered here have attracted international attention. The "Celluloid Angels" article has been referenced in a host of other publications and spawned a number of international radio interviews and commentary articles. Likewise, the "Celluloid Devils" article has been noted in various international publications and was awarded the Dr. Gene Tranbarger Writing Award in 2012 from the American Assembly of Men in Nursing. In qualitative analysis, stories matter, but only if we take the time to find the gems within them.

REFERENCES

Bayer, B. E. (2007). From angels to devils: Images of nurses in film. Retrieved from http://www.nursevillage.com/nv/content/personalside/entertainment

Burech, B., & Gordon, S. (2000). *From silence to voice*. Ithaca, NY: Cornell University Press.

Darbyshire, P., & Gordon, S. (2005). Exploring popular images and representations of nurses and nursing. In J. Daly, S. Speedy, D. Jackson, N. Lambert, & C. Lamberst (Eds.), *Professional nursing: Concepts, issues and challenges* (pp. 69–92). New York, NY: Springer Publishing.

Farella, C. (2001). Doormats, devils and divas: Nurses in the movies. Retrieved from http://news.nurse.com/appa/pbcs.dll/article?AID=2001101020316

Gordon, S., & Johnson R. (2004, March/April). How Hollywood portrays nurses: Report from the front row. *Revolution*, 15–21.

Herodotus, P. M. (1998). *The Histories* (first Rawlinson edition in 1858; J. M Dent, Ed.). London, UK: Orion Publishing Group.

Kalisch, B. J., & Kalisch, P. A. (1982). The image of the nurse in motion pictures. *American Journal of Nursing, 82*(4), 605–611.

Kalisch, B. J., Kalisch, P. A., & McHugh, M. L. (1982). The nurse as a sex object in motion pictures, 1930–1980. *Research in Nursing and Health, 5*, 147–154.

Polit, D. F., & Beck, C. T. (2012). *Nursing research: Generating and assessing evidence for nursing practice*. Wolter Kluwer/Lippincott Williams & Wilkins, Sydney.

Rasmussen, E. (2001). Picture imperfect: From Nurse Ratched to Hot Lips Houlihan, film/tv portrayals of nurses often transmit a warped image of real-life RNs. *NurseWeek*. May 7th.

Ritchie, J., & Lewis, J. (2003). *Qualitative research practice: A guide for social science students and researchers*. London, UK: Sage Publications.

Schneider, Z., Whitehead, D., LoBiondo-Wood, G., & Haber, J. (2013). *Nursing and midwifery research: Methods and appraisal for evidence-based practice* (4th ed.). Sydney, AU: Mosby/Elsevier.

Stanley, D. (2005). In command of care: Toward the theory of congruent leadership. *Journal of Research in Nursing, 11*(2), 132–144.

Stanley, D. (2006). In command of care: Clinical nurse leadership explored. *Journal of Research in Nursing, 11*(1), 20–39.

Stanley, D. (2008). Celluloid angels: A research study of nurses in feature films 1900–2007. *Journal of Advanced Nursing, 64*(1), 84–95.

Stanley, D. (2012). Celluloid devils: A research study of male nurses in feature films. *Journal of Advanced Nursing, 68*(11), 2526–2537.

Strauss, A., & Corbin, J. (1998). *Basics of qualitative research: Techniques and procedures for developing grounded theory*. London, UK: Sage Publications.

Walker, J. (2006). *Halliwell's: The only film guide that matters—Film, video & DVD guide 2007* (22nd ed.). London: HarperCollins.

Ward, C., Styles, I., & Bosco, A. (2003). Perceived status of nurses compared to other health care professionals. *Contemporary Nurse, 15*(1–2), 20–28.

CHAPTER SEVEN

THE NAVAJO EXPERIENCE OF ELIZABETH FORSTER, PUBLIC HEALTH NURSE

Mary Ann Ruffing-Rahal

PUBLIC HEALTH NURSING: CROSS-CULTURAL CORE

Long before the formal emergence of transcultural nursing in 1967, public health nurses had forged a tradition of effective cross-cultural liaisons between themselves and their clients/patients in both urban and rural settings (Leininger, 1967, 1970). From its inception in the 1880s, for example, organized community health nursing (visiting nursing) in the United States was a practice specialty with distinct cross-cultural foundations: Nurses worked to provide preventive, infectious disease, and maternal child services in the homes and neighborhoods of poor and immigrant populations in New York, Boston, Charleston, and other Eastern coastal cities. Henry Street Settlement House, founded by Lillian Wald and associates in 1893, became a symbol of the goals of the Progressive movement, which stressed activism and involvement in social issues on behalf of disenfranchised groups. Wald's singularly decisive influence on early public health nursing included her 1912 Red Cross initiative to institute a nationwide system of rural public health nursing, the Town and Country Nursing Service. Although short lived, this service nevertheless represented the expansion of public health nursing services to other culturally distinct yet remote populations (Buhler-Wilkerson, 1983, 1992; Clemen-Stone, Eigsti, & McGuire, 1991, pp. 10–14; Frachel, 1988; Sullivan, 1984).

Reprinted from Ruffing-Rahal, M. A. (1995). The Navajo experience of Elizabeth Forster, public health nurse. *Nursing History Review, 3*, 173–188. Copyright © 1995 by the American Association for the History of Nursing.

Early in the 20th century, Wald and other public health nursing leaders realized the benefits of advanced educational opportunities for their staffs, particularly for gaining a detailed understanding of sociocultural factors. They came to see that such knowledge was a necessary foundation to effective case finding and preventive education in culturally diverse populations. A small but important national movement, which originated at Teachers College, Columbia, and came to include various teachers' colleges and university departments of sociology/social work, promoted special educational programs for public health nurses (Clemen-Stone et al., 1991, p. 17). By the 1920s, Mary Breckinridge, a nurse–midwife with both clinical and graduate student experience in public health nursing, would organize the Frontier Nursing Service in the Kentucky Appalachian region, a family-centered health system with notable emphasis on its culturally distinct clientele (Dye, 1983; Ruffing-Rahal, 1990).

Evidence of the early cross-cultural core of public health nursing can be discerned from an examination of the clinical practice of Elizabeth Warham Forster, RN (1886–1972).[1] Born in Georgetown, South Carolina, she graduated from the nursing program at Baltimore's Union Memorial Hospital in 1912 and, subsequently, from an advanced course in public health nursing at Johns Hopkins University. In 1913, Forster moved to Colorado Springs, where she commenced professional employment with the Colorado Springs Visiting Nurses Association. By 1915, she was nursing supervisor.

During the flu outbreak of 1917, one of Forster's home nursing cases was a 26-year-old woman, Laura Gilpin, a native of Colorado Springs. Five years younger than Forster, Gilpin had studied photography in New York at the Clarence White School; she then embarked on an international career as a portrait and landscape photographer. Her illness and subsequent recuperation in Colorado Springs marked the beginning of a friendship between the women that would last over 50 years.

BACKGROUND

The *Dineh*, otherwise known as the Navajo people, were a common interest for Forster and Gilpin. The Dineh were the largest tribal group of Native American populations, and their reservation lands spanned the Four Corners area of Utah, Arizona, Colorado, and New Mexico (Wilson, 1983). Forster's and Gilpin's initial experience with the Navajo occurred in Arizona in the autumn of 1930, during a camping trip. Running out of gas in a desolate area, Gilpin left Forster with the car to hike several miles to the nearest trading post. Upon returning with help, Gilpin found Forster, whom she referred

Chapter 7. The Navajo Experience of Elizabeth Forster

to as Betsy, surrounded by Navajo people, all engrossed in playing cards on the hood of the automobile. There must have been a climate of immediate trust and rapport, as 1 year later, in November 1931, Forster accepted a position as field nurse for the New Mexico Association of Indian Affairs. She was assigned to an outpost situated in the Navajo community of Red Rock, Arizona, near the border with New Mexico, and would hold the position until April 1933. At the time, *field nurse* was the designated term for public health nurses employed within the Bureau of Indian Affairs (BIA; Gregg, 1965). Hired on the basis of her professional background in public health as well as for her camping skills, Forster was installed in an old mission hospital, and two rooms became both her private quarters and dispensary.

During Forster's employment with the Indian Service, Gilpin came for several extended visits. Gilpin's photographs captured glimpses of Forster's nursing style. Gilpin would accompany Forster on her daily nursing rounds, which consisted of visiting families in hogans, and would thereby gain the Dineh's acceptance of her "as the nurse's friend." Forster's entrée as a public health nurse within the Navajo community enabled Gilpin, equipped with her eight-by-ten large view camera and tripod, to witness at close range everyday Navajo life, including its ceremonies and rituals, and thus to produce a photodocument of the people and their lifestyle.

An excerpt from one of Forster's letters indicates the tacit sense of co-creation shared by the two women for the Navajo way of life:

> Homeward bound next day we stopped just at the foot of the mountains to pay a hogan visit. . . . The colorful costumes of the women and children gathered on the edge of the circle, the setting sun touching the yellow straw to golden glory in the foreground and the sky to a gorgeous curtain beyond, made a picture which Laura's camera couldn't resist, and I have another entry in my Navajo memories. (Forster, 1988, p. 109)

Forster felt the inadequacies of language as a vehicle to transmit the fullness of her experiences with the Navajo acutely and thus welcomed Gilpin's ability to supply photographic corroboration: "I long for the descriptive ability to show you the thing as I saw it . . . the cupping dome of the hogan with the fire glowing in the center, the group of blanketed figures seated on sheepskins close to the encircling wall, the dark faces which gleamed and faded as the fire flame leaped and died" (Forster, 1988, p. 126). Frequently, the two women used Gilpin's photographs as a vehicle to further their own understanding of Navajo customs and beliefs: "We spent several hours visiting this family. They were interested in us and in the things we observed.

They looked at every picture in my book with the greatest of interest, pointing out differences in costume, ornaments, or possessions. Then we watched the making of kneel-down bread. . . . It was very good" (Gilpin, 1968, p. 72).

After her employment at Red Rock, Forster planned to publish an account of her time with the Navajo, using edited letters to family and friends. However, these plans, which included collaborating with Gilpin as photographer, met with disappointing refusals from potential publishers over many years. Efforts were thwarted too by the Depression, World War II, and Forster's own declining health. Gilpin nevertheless was able to complete her photodocumentary classic, *The Enduring Navajo*, in 1968, which she warmly dedicated to Forster (Gilpin, 1968, p. v). She attributed her frontispiece and introductory photographs in the volume to early Navajo experiences with Forster (Gilpin, 1968, p. 23). Throughout her writings, Gilpin consistently acknowledged how Forster's nursing experience at Red Rock had given Gilpin the chance to witness firsthand the more intimate aspects of Dineh life:

> This intrepid friend of mine. . . . It is needless to say that it was only the remarkable place she made for herself in the lives of the Indians in this region that made it possible for me to make most of the pictures in this series. I was accepted as her friend and because of their trust in her (and hers in them), I was given many rare opportunities. I could add much to this story in telling of her work as I saw it during those visits. How the Indians found that they could always depend on her, how she mysteriously understood them in spite of a language barrier, her remarkable psychological understanding of them, her unerring judgment, her willingness to undergo real hardship to carry out her work, and above all, the feeling the Indians had for her. (Gilpin, 1968, p. 34)

Gilpin intensively recalled her experiences when Forster was field nurse in the chapter entitled "The Dineh," likewise reporting on Forster's "good judgment and skill" (Gilpin, 1968, p. 13) in a number of emergencies and noting for posterity those personal qualities that endeared Forster to the Navajo such as her "wonderful capacity for joking with a perfectly straight face" (Gilpin, 1968, p. 30).

NAVAJO RESERVATION

The context of health services on the Navajo Reservation during the early 1930s has been characterized as "the only time during the first half of the 20th century that the Indian Bureau even approached adequate staff levels"

(Raup, 1959). The settlement of Red Rock consisted of little more than a partly abandoned mission hospital and trading post. In 1931, Forster arrived on the reservation to find that no preparations had been made for her lodging, nor had necessary medical supplies arrived. She nevertheless began her tour of duty by driving about, surveying her assigned district in a "New Chevy" (Forster, 1988, p. 44). She traveled the lands spanning Santa Fe and Taos, meeting key representatives of the Indian Association situated in various locations and thereby gathering firsthand information regarding the customs, health care procedures, and contacts at the hospitals at Albuquerque, Laguna, and Shiprock. Forster was not to lose her sense of awe at the sight of the magnificent desert environment and red rock cliffs: "I cannot tell you how completely one loses one's sense of familiar identity and becomes imbued with the romance of ancient life which is suggested on every hand" (Forster, 1988, p. 43). Once personal quarters were established with furnishings and household items shipped from home, Forster initiated a custom of open hospitality to the surrounding Navajo: "My radio, goldfish, magazines, checkers, and cards attract guests almost every evening when I am at home, and Sunday is invariably full also" (Forster, 1988, p. 82). Refreshments served at Forster's table provided many with an initial venture in the domestic routines of the white Anglo culture.

Forster's letters reflect her perspective on Navajo culture from the vantage point of the trusted outsider, White woman, healer, and health care provider in an isolated, dwindling reservation town. She consciously viewed her circumstances as an opportunity to expand her understanding of and insight into Navajo life; she characterized the field nurse role as a "pioneering venture in Public Health Nursing amongst a strange people, which will present new and perplexing problems in health and psychology" (Forster, 1988, p. 38). As her time and affiliation with the Navajo increased, her understanding and appreciation of the culture deepened accordingly. She found politeness to be consistently their foremost characteristic. In her letters to friends and family, she captured in language such arresting visual icons of the culture as the Navajo hogan (Forster, 1988, p. 41), sand painting (Forster, 1988, p. 48), and the yeibichai dancers (Forster, 1988, p. 49).

Forster's letters also cataloged long days, a rigorous caseload, and an arduous environmental context. Supplementary duties included "dispensary supplies to be kept up, fresh solutions to be made, remedies compounded from drugs on hand, returned bottles to be sterilized and washed, and countless other small but necessary duties" (Forster, 1988, p. 108). She saw up to 200 patients monthly in hogan, dispensary, and clinic settings, all of which warranted travel time; she also took many trips transporting patients and families to the hospitals in Shiprock and Santa Fe: "It is hard to believe I have driven more than a thousand miles since I had the car greased in Santa Fe. I have estimated that my mileage is averaging over a hundred miles a day" (Forster, 1988, p. 97). When a typhoid epidemic struck in a neighboring district, Forster traveled a distance of 200 miles a day several times a week (Forster, 1988, p. 102).

Illnesses and conditions ranged from the chronic and long term to the imminently life-threatening: Trachoma, scabies, influenza, pneumonia, arthritis, frostbite, and toothache abounded. Because she did not speak the Navajo language, Forster soon enlisted a 22-year-old Navajo, Timothy Kellywood, to be her interpreter and assistant. Kellywood and his family became close friends of Forster as well as Gilpin. They also became cultural informants; Kellywood would pick up on current events happening on the reservation by going to the local trading post, and he would frequently accompany Forster on travels about the reservation, often in extreme weather. In winter, snowdrifts blocked the desert roads: "The trips to hogans and hospital are difficult and take an unbelievable amount of time owing to the condition of the roads. The snow is deep and badly drifted . . . and we get stuck and must dig the car out with exasperating frequency" (Forster, 1988, p. 57). Cold temperatures likewise were a signal for other special measures taken by Forster to encourage Navajo attendance at the clinics:

> The weather is so cold and my people have come from such distances that I am preparing and serving soup for them, and in my dispensary, warmed by a cheerful wood fire and advertising my soup in odoriferous fashion, is a popular place on clinic day. (Forster, 1988, p. 65)

In summertime, when the Navajo moved their families and sheep to the mountains, Forster walked or rode horseback, always with the possibility of a sudden storm, road washout, or sandstorm:

> When the wind blows, driving the sand before it in clouds, only necessity drags us from within doors. Sometimes it blows for days at a time with diabolic fury and persistence, and the strain on our nerves is tense beyond belief. Nevertheless, she held camp clinics and other routine activities, such as honoring the frequent requests of Medicine Men for "knosaze"/cough medicine. (Forster, 1988, p. 106)

Forster used her scant leisure time to focus on coordinating youth games and sports for Navajo boys and girls. She frequently made long drives in bad weather, transporting the youth to and from Santa Fe and Shiprock. Perceiving that boys adapted less readily than girls to Navajo hogan life after reservation school, Forster encouraged Kellywood to organize and coach a basketball team, which they subsequently managed together, driving the team as far as Colorado Springs for 4 days of basketball (Forster, 1988, p. 129).

CROSS-CULTURAL STRENGTHS

One can infer from specific accounts in her letters Forster's therapeutic presence among the Navajo was essentially that of a respectful witness committed to upholding Navajo customs, including their healing rites and rituals. Forster did not impose Western ways; she often participated as an adjunct to, instead of a substitute for, the Navajo healing system. For example, Forster described her complementary role at a delivery in a hogan:

> I was . . . allowed to do the umbilical dressing and rub the wee one with oil after which I was firmly bidden to hold it over a trough of sand prepared on the hogan floor while an attendant poured first cold then warm water over the little body, and the old lady rubbed it vigorously . . . the result was a fresh pink-tan baby. (Forster, 1988, p. 96)

Cultural brokerage, represented by efforts to translate, bridge, negotiate, and link Navajo and Western medical cultures, was thus the foundation of Forster's nursing process (Tripp-Reimer & Brink, 1985). Her style as a culture broker was fully manifest in her account of the burial of an elderly woman:

> Timothy and I . . . collected some old planks, sawed them the proper length for a coffin, put them in the car with hammer and nails, and set out. Arrived at the old woman's home we nailed the box together and were ready to proceed. . . . When our undertaking duties were accomplished we were ready to prepare the grave. After some conversation with the family Timothy announced that they wished to bury her in the hogan but feared I might object since they knew it was contrary to white custom. Knowing that the hogan in which death has occurred is invariably deserted and never used again, I saw no reason for objection—in fact I rather approved the sentiment—So Timothy and the son-in-law began the difficult task of digging a grave in the hard-packed hogan floor. When it was finally deep enough to serve we managed to

get the box in, and then . . . to my vast amazement and utter horror, the family (much too well informed of white custom) requested me to "say something." . . . My bedazed brain leapt wildly from "Now I Lay Me" to "Dust Thou Art to Dust returneth was not written of the Soul," and I finally managed to ask the two English speaking members of the congregation if they could say the Lord's Prayer. They were reassuringly doubtful so I announced that we would say it anyway. The box was then covered with sheepskins and the grave filled. Then came the nailing up of the hogan door, the closing of the opening in the top, and our old lady was left to rest in the home where she had spent happy years. (Forster, 1988, pp. 86–87)

Exchange, a pattern consistently revealed in Forster's accounts of her interpersonal relations, included instances with Forster in the role of recipient:

Some time ago I decided that I would get my friends to teach me to card, spin, and weave as all Navajo women do, thinking that they would be readier to learn some things from me if they were teaching me something in return. So I bought wool from the Trader, washed it carefully and am now trying to learn to card. Each of my friends has to show me her own particular method and must laugh at my awkward efforts. (Forster, 1988, p. 82)

Similarly, Forster's visits sometimes included tangible items such as the "gift of fruit which the old man loves" (Forster, 1988, p. 135). In return for her nursing services, she received items such as lamb, potatoes and other crops, or rugs and artifacts. Occasionally, there came the gift of friendship: "Mary . . . to my surprise (I hadn't suspected friendship there) . . . shyly presented me with a nice ring" (Forster, 1988, p. 79). Forster's nonimposing nature was reflected in an account of a visit to an acutely ill elderly man, who was unwilling to be hospitalized, in his hogan:

Early in the morning . . . I set out at once and found the man badly in need of hospitalization, although unwilling . . . to go. . . . Argument and persuasion, reason, logic and warning are alike unavailing with the Navajos in the matter of illness (which they always think is due to the influence of chindis or evil spirits), so after doing what I could and explaining what relief he might expect from hospital treatment, I left with the assurance I would take him in to the hospital any time he decided to go. (Forster, 1988, p. 115)

The Navajo came to refer to her as *Asdzaa Bahozhoni*, which meant "The Happy One," a testament to her approachable demeanor. Moreover, one elderly woman affectionately addressed her as "Shedazy" or "Little Sister" (Forster, 1988, p. 103).

In blending healing elements from the cultures of both Navajo and Western medicine, Forster's practice incorporated both cooperative and collaborative elements (Spector, 1991). Forster's presence in the Navajo community was that of a friendly and trustworthy outsider throughout her tenure as field nurse; as Forster gained trust among the Dineh, she eventually was invited to participate in some of the Navajo healing rituals. While most of her interventions, representing the cooperative mode, were separate and distinct from those of the Navajo healers and occurred during hogan visits and dispensary hours, as well as in outreach clinics, her letters recount instances of collaborative practice with the medicine men. Here Forster joins a Navajo healer in a healing ceremony for an elder:

> He held up both hands with fingers folded, except the two forefingers which he placed side by side to show how we would work together. I sat and watched him as he sang and the earnest kindness of the face with its closed eyes and serious expression was impressive, and the monotonous clink of his deer hoof rattle soothing. (Forster, 1988, p. 123)

On another occasion, Forster took her medicine bag and held a clinic outside the hogan where a medicine man was conducting a sand painting ceremony. Ultimately, it was her identity among the Navajo as a healer that proved most satisfying. "Almost more interesting than any I have had before" (Forster, 1988, p. 125).

> I waited while Timothy went into the hogan, where the Medicine Man was singing, to ask if I might enter. He returned with permission and I went in. As I entered some one made a remark which was greeted with laughter. I knew, of course, that it was at my expense, but it sounded good natured and I was sure it was not offensive. Timothy told me afterwards that the remark had been Oh, this is one of our own medicine men, so it is all right. The idea that I am a medicine man and at their service is a source of kindly amusement to them always. (Forster, 1988, p. 125)

Forster perceived herself foremost as the advocate of and for the Navajo people, expressing with special intensity her earnest and unceasing efforts to increase personal "understanding [of] . . . the suffering and needs of my Navajo neighbors. The things we would consider the barest and poorest necessities would spell more than comfort and luxury to them. My food and shelter, coat and coal, begin to hurt and weigh upon my spirits. What can I do to help them?" (Forster, 1988, p. 64).

Forster did not present herself in any didactic or absolute manner. Instead, openness and self-evaluation were consistent aspects of her approach to the Navajo people. On one occasion, for example, she reflected candidly in a letter that she might have reacted less judgmentally to alcohol consumption on the reservation. In many instances, she was able to transcend cultural differences by means of her interpersonal brightness and wit:

> John . . . is evidently suffering . . . from the flu and I thought it wise to take him to the doctor for an examination. He demurred, but I told him I intended to take him if I had to use a rope. He laughed at this and repeated it to his wife. . . . I have fallen in love with her. Her face is very expressive and she has a happy sense of humor. When John . . . went into his hogan to prepare to accompany me she followed him and presently appeared leading him on a rope which she handed to me. The giggles which we enjoyed together over this joke sealed our friendship. (Forster, 1988, p. 80)

CONFLICT

Forster increasingly pondered the hardships and inequities ingrained in the reservation way of life for the Navajo:

> A period like this when hardship and want, discomfort and suffering press close around me stirs my mind to unhappy wonder. Whose the fault? These people really do live in the same land of plenty with their white "brothers." Time was, no doubt, when their own portion of this wielded as generous a living as they know but a great increase in numbers and no space or chance for expansion have resulted in a pitiful paucity of living requisites. The Navajo, as are other Indians in New Mexico and Arizona, are wards of our Government. Does that not mean that our Government is responsible for their welfare? Must they live in such discomfort as would surely distress the most callous? Must they die each winter from cold and hunger? As I sit by the fire and listen to the voice of the bitter wind I wonder at the blitheness of spirit that has filled our pleasant weather. (Forster, 1988, p. 92)

Her loyalty to Navajo integrity and autonomy was frequently challenged and undermined by the contrasting goals and initiatives of the two major bureaucracies in Navajo Reservation life: The Anglo church and the BIA. The local missionary had been a source of irritation for Forster from her earliest days at Red Rock, attempting to accompany Forster on her visits to hogans and capitalizing on her trusted access to families:

> To my consternation the Missionary finds this an opportunity to spread the Gospel and accompanies me with Bible and hymn book, and my nursing visit becomes a hogan prayer meeting. I listen as he "tells the story" and find it bewildering even without the complication of interpretation and am sure that by the time . . . the . . . interpreter has rendered his version it must be entirely incomprehensible to the Navajo. Apparently knowing nothing of the faith they seek to destroy, some of these determined Mission workers term it devil worship and superstition, and yet fail utterly to present Christianity in a form which primitive minds might grasp. (Forster, 1988, p. 51)

Forster also criticized the reservation boarding schools established by the BIA and their long-term hazardous effects on Navajo culture:

> They have learned to live by standards impossible to hogan life, have been taught to regard their fathers' religion as superstition, failing meanwhile to grasp the meaning of Christianity, have apparently small chance and less incentive to make use of the education thus acquired, and so, present a picture of idle, useless youth. (Forster, 1988, p. 128)

Conflict arose amidst a number of stressful circumstances in 1933. Timothy, her trusted assistant, received what she perceived as an unfair sentence by the Navajo court and spent time in jail (Forster, 1988, pp. 132–134). Also, the nationwide Depression was impacting negatively on the funding of nursing programs within the New Mexico Association on Indian Affairs, resulting in delayed payment of monthly salaries (Sandweiss, 1988, pp. 13–15). As the most recently hired staff member, Forster struggled over whether to leave and thus alleviate some of the financial burden. Further, the local Indian Affairs agent neglected to deliver Forster's winter coat and likewise redesignated her dispensary space a dining room, thus leaving her without the practice setting familiar to her clients (Forster, 1988, pp. 138).

Sandweiss, Forster's editor, reports that Forster faced an ultimate moral dilemma at this time: She had to choose whether to side with the local Indian Affairs superintendent and physician at Shiprock in condemning the medicine man as evil, thereby intending to discredit his power and authority among the Navajo, or whether to uphold her belief in the Navajo healing tradition (Forster, 1988, pp. 138–140; Sandweiss, 1988, pp. 13–16). Of course, Forster was too steadfast an advocate of Navajo autonomy, dignity, and wisdom to condemn the Navajo healers. At the same time, she realized that the always tenuous foundations of support for her position as field nurse had irrefutably disintegrated. Following an ambivalent resignation, Forster departed Red Rock in April 1933. Gilpin arrived in time to help Forster pack her belongings and was with her on the last morning as she said goodbye to loyal Navajo friends. Although Forster and Gilpin would return several times to the reservation, Forster's tenure as Navajo field nurse was over. The Navajo did commission a letter, written in English and directed to the New Mexico Health Service, protesting the loss of their field nurse (Sandweiss, 1988, pp. 16–18).

In the sadness and disillusionment following her departure from Red Rock, Forster realized the short-term and tenuous nature of her total effort with the Navajo people:

> It is a keen interest in their development which makes us loath to leave them. My small contribution to their comfort does not really matter. Individuals are born, suffer and die and the life of a race is not much affected by the alleviation of suffering in a few or the saving of a few lives. It is education which vitally affects the future, and one wishes it might be more intelligently directed. (Forster, 1988, pp. 140)

DISCUSSION

Cultural discrimination and crisis pervade many contemporary realities of health care. As the cultural contexts of health and illness continue to be explored, there is renewed interest in cultural theory and processes, especially as realized and embodied in real world practitioners. To this end, published accounts of practice experience in specialties such as nurse midwifery (Armstrong & Feldman, 1986; Breckinridge, 1981) and public health nursing (Milio, 1970) remain invaluable as a source of insight into and validation of cultural themes. The published letters of Elizabeth Forster make a contribution with their detailed portrayal of the cross-cultural context of public health nursing on the Navajo reservation.

In her own letters and through the photographic/literary work of Gilpin, Elizabeth Forster provides a compelling early example of the culturally aware health care provider. Forster reported on the dynamics of culture, environment, and health in her written accounts to friends and family. In her nursing practice, Forster was adventurous, sensitive, and intelligent. Forster was clearly disappointed by the turn of events at Red Rock; realizing her own professional powerlessness, she perceived its parallel in the continuing interplay of manipulation and devaluation of the Navajo by local representatives of Christianity, Western medicine, and the U.S. government.

One might have anticipated that Forster, after electing to leave her treasured roles as health care provider and healer among the Navajo, would continue efforts as an advocate on behalf of culturally appropriate political and social change on the reservation. This, however, was not the case for Forster, who lived another four decades, frequently in poor health and in varying circumstances.

After first leaving the reservation, Forster and Gilpin, in their wish to depict the culture as they had been privileged to experience it firsthand, planned a book of edited letters about the Navajo. Although Forster did assemble her letters as a prelude to securing a publishing contract, the collaborative work envisioned by the two never did materialize. Nevertheless, the image of public health nursing that can be deciphered from Forster's selected letters and that is reinforced by the writing and photographs of Laura Gilpin reflects an exemplar of enthusiasm, compassionate care, and advocacy for the Navajo way of life. Considering their visual and verbal texts as a co-created unit, the work of Forster and Gilpin provides a compelling and poignant vignette of some of the realities of public health nursing practice, bygone and imminent.

ACKNOWLEDGMENT

The author wishes to acknowledge the clerical assistance of Michelle Compston and Patty Egger.

NOTE

1. Content analysis was carried out on two published primary sources of autobiographic writing. First, 37 of Forster's edited letters, written between September 1931 and May 1933 (her time on the reservation), are incorporated, along with

some of Gilpin's photographs, from Forster (1988). Of Forster's 37 letters, one is to an unnamed recipient. Otherwise, 15 letters were written to Laura Gilpin, 11 to Forster's younger sister, and the remaining 10 to two women friends. For the second primary source, autobiographic description and photographs contained in Gilpin (1968) were examined for potential illustration and enlargement of themes in Forster's letters. The letters of Elizabeth Forster were among the papers of Laura Gilpin bequeathed in 1979 to the Amon Carter Museum in Fort Worth, Texas, where they subsequently were discovered, and are quoted by permission of Jerry Richardson and the Amon Carter Museum.

REFERENCES

Armstrong, P., & Feldman, S. (1986). *A midwife's story*. New York, NY: Arbor House.
Breckinridge, M. (1981). *Wide neighborhoods: A story of the Frontier Nursing Service*. Lexington, KY: University Press of Kentucky.
Buhler-Wilkerson, K. (1983). False dawn: The rise and decline of public health nursing in America, 1900–1930. In E. C. Lagemann (Ed.), *Nursing history: New perspectives, new possibilities* (pp. 89–106). New York, NY: Teachers College Press.
Buhler-Wilkerson, K. (1992). Caring in its proper place: Race and benevolence in Charleston, SC, 1813–1930. *Nursing Research, 41*, 14–20.
Clemen-Stone, S., Eigsti, D. G., & McGuire, S. L. (1991). *Comprehensive family and community health nursing* (3rd ed.). St. Louis, MO: C.V. Mosby.
Dye, N. S. (1983). Mary Breckinridge: The Frontier Nursing Service and the introduction of nurse-midwifery in the United States. *Bulletin of the History of Medicine, 57*, 485–507.
Forster, E. W. (1988). *Denizens of the desert: A tale in word and picture of life among the Navajo Indians* (M. A. Sandweiss, Ed.). Albuquerque, NM: University of New Mexico Press.
Frachel, R. R. (1988). A new profession: The evolution of public health nursing. *Public Health Nursing, 5*, 86–90.
Gilpin, L. (1968). *The enduring Navajo*. Austin, TX: University of Texas Press.
Gregg, E. D. (1965). *The Indians and the nurse*. Norman, OK: University of Oklahoma Press.
Leininger, M. (1967). The cultural concept and its relevance to nursing. *Journal of Nursing Education, 6*(4), 27–39.
Leininger, M. (1970). *Nursing and anthropology: Two worlds to blend*. New York, NY: John Wiley & Sons.
Milio, N. (1970). *9226 Kercheval: The storefront that did not burn*. Ann Arbor, MI: University of Michigan Press.
Raup, R. (1959). *The Indian health program from 1800–1955*. Washington, DC: U.S. Department of Health, Education, and Welfare, Public Health Service.
Ruffing-Rahal, M. A. (1990). Ethnographic traits in the writing of Mary Breckinridge. *Journal of Advanced Nursing, 16*, 614–620.

Sandweiss, M. A. (Ed.). (1988). Introduction. In *Denizens of the desert: A tale in word and picture of life among the Navajo Indians*. Albuquerque, NM: University of New Mexico Press.
Spector, R. E. (1991). *Cultural diversity in health and illness* (3rd ed.). Norwalk, CT: Appleton & Lange.
Sullivan, J. (1984). *Directions in community health nursing*. Boston, MA: Blackwell Scientific Publications.
Tripp-Reimer, T., & Brink, P. J. (1985). Culture brokerage. In G. M. Bulechek & J. C. McCloskey (Eds.), *Nursing interventions: Treatments for nursing diagnosis* (pp. 352–364). Philadelphia, PA: W. B. Saunders.
Wilson, U. M. (1983). Nursing care of American Indian patients. In M. S. Orque, B. Bloch, & L. S. A. Monroy (Eds.), *Ethnic nursing care: A multicultural approach* (pp. 271–295). St. Louis, MO: C. V. Mosby.

CHAPTER EIGHT

SOJOURNER: LIFE STORIES OF A GLOBAL HEALTH NURSE

Barbara A. Anderson

Ten years old seems terribly old when one is 10. Shortly after my birthday, as the languid summer days shortened and the dreaded beginning of the school year approached, I decided it was time to write down my life goals. In the garden of my rural Midwestern home, I wrote my goals—to see the whole world and to have six children (after seeing the whole world, of course). The world seemed simple and possible. I concluded that the way to see the whole world was to pursue my desire, since age 4, to become a nurse. Then I would employ my healing skills on a boat down the Nile, saving sick babies. Some of these babies I would adopt, and someday I would give birth to a few children. These were the dreams of a child whose childhood would soon come to an abrupt end. Life has not been as simple as I envisioned in the garden many years ago. It would leave scars, each one weaving the tapestry of a journey.

REFUGEE HERITAGE

My life is textured in stories of refugees. My mother's family were Irish and Russian immigrants. In 1856, among those emigrating in rickety ships from the southern coast of Ireland was a 9-year-old named John Rooney and his parents. Refugees from the devastating Irish potato famine, they landed in New York and made their way to Illinois. In 1861, at the age of 14, heeding the call to arms from President Abraham Lincoln, John enlisted as a Yankee

---

This chapter is an excerpt from the author's memoir: Anderson, B. (2013). *A life apart: Stories of a sojourner*. St. Louis, MO: Mira Publishing. Published with permission of author.

soldier. After an honorable discharge in 1865, John returned to civilian life and married, thus beginning my Irish American lineage. Shortly after the Civil War, in the wake of severe religious persecution, a wealthy Jewish family left their czarist Russian homeland, migrating to America. Their son, Clarence, and John Rooney's daughter, Ellen, were my grandparents. They eloped as their union was strongly opposed by both her Roman Catholic family and his Orthodox Jewish family. My mother was the youngest of their four children. The oldest child died of scarlet fever at age 5. My grandmother never recovered from losing this child. She began hearing voices, seeing visions, and sliding into insanity. She became increasingly abusive to my mother, culminating in life-threatening violence. All her life, my mother would suffer from flashbacks of this abuse.

When my mother was 14, my grandmother was committed to an "insane asylum." My grandfather disappeared, never seen again. Shortly afterwards, my grandmother died mysteriously in a suspected beating episode in the hospital. My mother spent the next 10 years with her older sister and husband. An excellent student, she dreamed of being a nurse. She was accepted into a diploma school of nursing, but she had no money. Her older sister and brother-in-law, quite wealthy from his business, refused to loan her the money. They reasoned she would be more useful working in their retail business. She was brokenhearted, always retaining the desire to be a nurse. A few years later, she met and eloped with my father.

My father's family also came to America as refugees, but at a much earlier date. In 1642, England erupted into religious oppression and violence. In the wake of this civil war, a new religious sect, the Society of Friends, was founded. The guiding force was George Fox, a man of deep conviction about the power of the Spirit, pacifism, and the inner light in each person. The small sect grew rapidly, generating concern among traditional religious forces. A name of derision for this new sect, "Quaker," was bestowed upon George Fox in 1650 during a court trial. Fox had admonished the prosecuting magistrate to "tremble at the word of the Lord." The magistrate responded by bestowing a name of ridicule upon the sect—Quakers (Bacon, 1999).

The Society of Friends became a formidable force, attracting educated and influential followers. Among them was William Penn, the son of an influential man in the English court. Seeking to rid himself of this troublemaker, King Charles II granted Penn's proposal for a land grant in the American colonies. In 1682, Penn launched his "holy experiment" in Pennsylvania, a place of refuge for persons persecuted for their faith (Bacon, 1999). Even today, the Society of Friends is a global leader in providing sanctuary to refugees.

My ancestor, Robert Hodgson, was born in England in 1675. He became an officer in the British army, where he became acquainted with and joined the Society of Friends. He married an English woman and they had three children. They fled religious persecution, sailing from Ireland in 1710. An epidemic raged throughout the ship, killing the entire family except for one child, George. He was adopted and raised by a Quaker family in Philadelphia. At age of 28, George married an American-born Quakeress, and they had six children.

Persecution of the Quakers continued on both sides of the Atlantic. Peter Stuyvesant, governor of "New York," the Dutch territory in the American colonies, waged a war of brutal persecution against the Quakers in Pennsylvania. The historical document, *New England Judged by the Spirit of the Lord* (Bishop, 1661), relates the torture and harassment of the Quakers. In 1751, George and his family, seeking respite from the ongoing persecutions, joined other Quakers migrating to North Carolina. There they and their descendants lived in peace until the Civil War loomed and the issue of slavery became a national debate. The Quakers were pacifists, refusing to hold slaves. The Quakers in the South were especially harassed, their crops and animals destroyed, their barns and homes burned (Bacon, 1999). Word from Quakers in the free territories in the Ohio Valley spoke of fertile agriculutural rich land and prohibition of slavery.

North Carolina Quakers Levi and Catherine Coffin had organized the "Underground Railroad," a well-orchestrated communication line for clandestine movement of escaping slaves from the South to Canada. In 1826 Coffin and his family migrated to Indiana, settling on land adjacent to the Ohio River. The Coffin family led the Underground Railroad movement from their home. One December night, a barefooted woman carrying her baby appeared at their door. She was on the edge of death, having fled across the frozen river. The Coffins saved her life, along with 2000 other slaves. The flight of Eliza is a key story that Quaker author Harriet Beecher Stowe, friend of the Coffins and the Hodgsons, told in the book *Uncle Tom's Cabin* (Stowe, 1852). Written in the decade before the Civil War, this book polarized the nation.

If a runaway slave could get across the Ohio River, there was hope for freedom, although slavers and their posses frequently searched for hidden slaves on Quaker farms. Although buying and selling slaves was illegal in the free territories, recovering "contraband," escaped slaves, was not. The 1793 Fugitive Slave Act made it compulsory for all citizens to assist in apprehending runaways. Quaker families used passive resistance in defying this law. They refused to release or even acknowledge the presence of runaway slaves on their farms (Bacon, 1999). Legend has it that one Quaker faced down a posse, saying, "There are no slaves here, for in God's eyes no man is a slave." The posse left empty-handed.

In the summer of 1831, the entire Guilford county North Carolina Quaker community, including the Hodgson family, sold their properties and traveled by wagon to the Ohio Valley. They bought land in western Indiana, refusing the land that President Andrew Jackson had forcefully taken from native Americans and offered to settlers as land grant property. The Hodgson family worked with the Coffin family, coordinating the Underground Railroad on the western side of the state. For unknown reasons, they changed their family name to Hodson. My ancestor, Joel, an adolescent at the time, chronicled the migration to the Ohio Valley and captured the story of the Hodson participation in the historical Underground Railroad movement. The barn on the family farm, with a removable bottom floor, was the hiding place for slaves. When runaway slaves, crouching below a load of hay, arrived at the farm, the Hodson family fed, clothed, and hid them until the next route north could be arranged. Generations later, I took my children on a family pilgrimage of the Underground Railroad starting at the historical Coffin home on the Ohio River and culminating at our ancestral home.

The ensuing generations of Hodsons farmed the fertile land. They battled many assaults on health, including recurrent epidemics of streptococcal erysipelas. Antibiotics would have saved their lives, but the miracle drugs were not discovered for another century. Maternal mortality was a constant threat to the women. The blessing of dependable family planning would not arrive until 180 years later when Margaret Sanger, nurse, public health advocate, and founder of Planned Parenthood, collaborated with Dr. John Rock, fertility specialist, in implementing the clinical trials on the birth control pill (BCP). The BCP was tested, not only in Mexico where the initial plant source was discovered, but also in Appalachia, under the direction of Mary Breckinridge, public health nurse, nurse–midwife, and founder of the frontier nursing service (FNS; Breckinridge, 1952). The BCP would prove to be life-saving for millions of women.

Infant mortality was also high. My twin aunts were born at home in 1904, attended by an untrained country doctor. The first child emerged a robust baby; the undiagnosed twin "died aborning," strangling on her umbilical cord. Such calamities are avoidable with well-prepared health care professionals. During this period, the Flexner report was exposing the gross inadequacies in medical education, and concurrently, in England, Florence Nightingale was setting the standards for professional nursing. The people of Indiana, the Hoosiers, relied upon traditional remedies described in the book *Hoosier Home Remedies* (Tyler, 1985). As children, my siblings and I were frequently subjected to these traditional remedies: pipe smoke blown into an aching ear or sassafras tea for a stomach ache. My grandmother dug sassafras roots from our backyard tree, brewing them into a foul-tasting tea. The "rheumatiz" was a common affliction during the damp, bone-chilling winters. One neighbor described a favorable outcome after dosing her arthritic husband with traditional herbs. She stated, "It done him a power of good."

My grandparents raised three children during the "roaring twenties" and the Great Depression. My father was the youngest of this eighth generation of Hodson immigrants. I grew up listening to stories of Quaker refugees, the Underground Railroad, and the Great Depression, as my grandmother and I sewed. Sewing was a valued skill taught to young girls as soon as they could hold a needle. Much later as a nurse–midwifery student, while learning to suture, my preceptor remarked, "You must have learned to sew as a child. You do this with complete ease."

During the lifetime of my parents, the world was rapidly changing. Radio brought the world to rural America. World War I raged and ended; the Spanish flu killed millions; automobiles replaced horses; and the Ku Klux Klan harassed Black sharecroppers. My grandfather told me stories about the Ku Klux Klan. He described their midnight visits to the log cabins of Black freedmen and to his childhood home. The Klan burned crosses in front of their homes and lynched some of the Black population. These stories always haunted me. One summer my parents, siblings, and I took a road trip to the South. We piled into our old car, camping through Appalachia and on the beaches in Florida. We returned through the back country of the Deep South. Prior to the Civil Rights Movement and sheltered by our Quaker community, we were naïve to the poisons of racial hatred. I had heard the stories of the Ku Klux Klan from my grandfather, but they seemed like stories from a past era. The oppression and segregation in rural Southern towns was very present. It burned into my consciousness.

Many years later, I was a university professor in California. Proposition 87 was a ballot initiative on the California slate, aimed at denying health benefits or education for undocumented immigrants, mostly Mexican and Central Americans. This proposed ban included children and pregnant women. Health professionals and public school teachers in California went on record opposing the proposition. I was asked to speak against the proposition. I requested that my graduate students in public health attend, as they were learning about political advocacy. The organizers of the rally agreed. Just as the students and I left for the rally, my phone rang. The police informed me that the Ku Klux Klan, supporting the proposition, had named me as the target of a death threat. The police cautioned that Klan members had already assembled at the site and security was insufficient. The county sheriff ordered the rally stopped. The Klan won that round, and the initiative was passed in California. There was outrage and threats of civil disobedience. The initiative was never implemented and remains in appeal in the California legal system.

A MIDWESTERN CHILDHOOD

My father was a gifted man, earning a college scholarship in chemistry. When he graduated, he took a short train trip to the upper Midwest. There he met my mother on a blind date. It was instant chemistry, and my parents eloped 6 weeks later. My urban Roman Catholic mother moved to a rural Quaker farming community. It has always amazed me how tolerant my parents were of each other's cultural and religious backgrounds. Just as they married, Pearl Harbor was attacked, pivoting America into World War II.

After World War II my father was released from government service. I suddenly appeared, quickly followed by four siblings. My parents longed for their children to have a place to run, explore, and feel connections. They settled in a small Indiana town, a former Underground Railroad station. Our home was a marvelous place to be a kid in, a one-acre property with a large, sprawling clapboard house and a horse barn. The best part of the house was the basement, dark and spooky, where we created imaginary friends and ghosts, the most memorable being the "crimson ghost." The neighborhood was very safe. With no regard for all the frightful things that could have happened, we biked, swam, skated, and explored with abandon. In the evenings, my father played his beloved baby grand piano, the pure ivory keys ringing out love songs he had written for our mother. At age 4, I decided to become a nurse and, in preparation, regularly patched up fallen and scraped siblings and neighborhood kids.

Sometimes I would sneak away during the summer months to lie on the hill above the Mexican migrant workers' camp, watching these fascinating people go about their lives. They came to work in the fields, planting and harvesting the bountiful Midwestern tomato crop. I loved the sound of their language. Finally I mustered the courage to approach the camp, finding that the people were friendly, spoke a little English, and offered me a new food (a tortilla). Over time, I got to know these families. One day, they told me that one of the field workers, a young woman about 16 years old, was lying in an adjacent, abandoned barn, having just given birth. I ran home to tell my mother. When I got home, my mother said, "Where *were* you this time?"

"Mom," I said. "Please, just listen." Hearing my description and without a moment's hesitation, she gathered blankets, baby clothes, and clean cloths. We hiked into that muddy camp where she bathed the young mother and baby and gave her money to see the local doctor, who pronounced both mother and baby fit and healthy. That was one of the most powerful experiences of my childhood. That is when I knew my nursing career would focus on mothers and babies, but it took another experience to know that I was called to be a midwife. We had a succession of mutt dogs but my favorite was our beautiful border collie, Lassie. Hers was the first birth I "attended." Lying on my bed all night, Lassie had gentle contractions. Suddenly, she stood up, delivering five perfect little puppies into my very soggy bed. She had trouble breaking one of the amniotic sacs which I tore with my fingernail. That was a defining moment. I knew that I would care for mothers and babies around the time of birth.

From the time I was 5 my mother's health deteriorated. Her nutrition was poor, she was a heavy smoker, she had five pregnancies quickly, and she struggled with flashbacks of her childhood abuse. No real effort was made to find out why her health was so poor until she discovered a lump in her left breast. My parents questioned whether the diethylstilbestrol injections she had received with the last three pregnancies caused the cancer. In those days, diethylstilbestrol was given as "prevention" for miscarriage (although she never had any signs of impending miscarriages). The conventional wisdom, later disputed, was that diethylstilbestrol played no role in promoting breast cancer. Mom was stricken with grief, fear, and pain. With her history of abuse, she had limited defenses, and there was no therapy for these problems. The cancer rapidly spread to her right breast. Our Quaker community provided the practical aid that has been their legacy. An African American friend, Cassie, who was a housekeeper for a wealthy family, helped us clean the house whenever my father could afford it. When my father paid Cassie, she always slipped into the bedroom to say good-bye to our very sick mother. Once I heard her say, "Now, honey, you just keep this money and let me know the next time you need a cleaning." When I was in high school, one of Cassie's twin girls died suddenly from a ruptured atrial-venous malformation. My mother handed me an envelope with a lot of cash. She had saved all the money that Cassie had returned to her. "Take this to Cassie," she said. "They are going to need this for the funeral." How like the O. Henry's story, *The Gift of the Magi* (O. Henry, Reprint 2001).

As my mother was dying, my father and I took turns changing the bandages covering necrotic wounds. One afternoon, the cancer eroded through an artery and blood spurted everywhere. I stuck my finger directly into the artery and twisted it to stop the bleeding. After that incident, the family doctor arranged for us to have daily nursing care in the home. Janet was our nurse. With her hand on my shoulder, she told me I was doing a good job of bandaging the gaping, cancerous holes. I wanted to be like Janet. June 24, 1963, dawned a perfect summer morning. My father and I had been up most of the night caring for my mother. Janet arrived, telling us to take a break. We both hugged my mother, telling her we loved her. I've always thought that my mother chose that moment to leave. Janet went into the bedroom and then motioned to my father. A few minutes later, he came out and gathered me in his arms, asking me to explain to my siblings that mother was gone. The Quaker community sprang into action. Food began to arrive. One "friend" stopped by to see if she could help, spotted a huge load of laundry by the washing machine, and scooped it up. A few hours later, it was returned washed, folded and pressed. Our community was so good to us, but our world was shattered.

THE TOUGHEST JOB I EVER LOVED

The ensuing years were difficult. I studied nursing at Indiana University while helping my father with the family. In nursing school, I had two classmates, African exchange students, both on Fulbright scholarships completing their BSN degrees. Upon graduation, they returned to Africa to assume leadership positions. Samuel was from Uganda and Tenanya from Ethiopia. They encouraged me to fulfill my dream to come to Africa. Our paths would cross in the future.

Peace Corps was claiming the imagination of America's youth after President John Kennedy's call to action. My father encouraged me to follow my dream, and I applied, listing Africa as my first choice of assignment. I was ecstatic to receive my assignment to Ethiopia, in east Africa. The last semester of nursing school was a whirl as I prepared to take the nursing licensure exam and begin the 3-month Peace Corps language and cultural training at the University of California, Los Angeles (UCLA). I had only been out of Indiana once on the family camping trip, and I had never been on an airplane. As I write now, I have exceeded three million miles of air travel!

Peace Corps training was grueling, 12 hours each day of Amharic language training by Ethiopian nationals, graduate students at UCLA. If we wanted to eat, we had to ask for the food in Amharic! To pass the training phase, we had to demonstrate basic verbal proficiency by the end of the 3-month training period. Amharic is cognate with Hebrew, vastly different from English. Some Peace Corps volunteers (PCVs) of Jewish origin had closer familiarity with the language structure. Later, on annual leave from Ethiopia, I toured Israel. My cheap suitcase had broken, and I tried to bargain for a new bag in English and limited French. The market vendor in Tel Aviv tried German, Greek, and Turkish. We were at a stalemate. Finally, remembering the historic links between Hebrew and Amharic, I tried Amharic. The vendor broke into a huge grin, replied in Hebrew, and the deal was struck.

There were 60 PCV trainees in my Ethiopia training group, 15 of them nurses in the health training cohort. Seven weeks into our training, we were called into a meeting with an officer from Peace Corps headquarters in Washington, D.C. This officer was Nina Rusk, RN, cousin of Secretary of State Dean Rusk. A warm and savvy global health nurse, she informed us that the Peace Corps had selected our health cohort to be the first trainees in the history of the Peace Corps to experiment with "in-country training." Instead of completing our training at UCLA, we were to leave for Ethiopia almost immediately to conclude our training on site. The focus of the training would be a 1-month tour circling Ethiopia, learning about rural primary health care, the regional hospital system, and the key health conditions in the country: malaria, tuberculosis, schistosomiasis, smallpox, kwashiorkor, marasmus, infant diarrhea, and maternal health problems. Nina and her Ethiopian nurse colleagues would orient us; we would continue our language training on the bus between sites; and we would conduct rural mobile clinics.

The pressure was on. The health cohort had to pass the Amharic language testing at two-thirds basic proficiency, 7 weeks into the training program. We were subjected to an accelerated schedule of vaccinations and issued passports. We flew to our homes for 3 days to say good-bye to our families and to gather our belongings (with a limited luggage weight of 100 pounds for 2 years of service). The Peace Corps assured us that we would have books from the Peace Corps library in Addis Ababa, the capital of Ethiopia, but not professional textbooks. I used most of my packing weight for my textbooks, a good decision because resources were very limited in Ethiopia. When I finished Peace Corps service, I left all those books with the nursing school where I had taught. In my 3 years of Peace Corps service, I reread (and in some cases, read!) those textbooks cover to cover on dark nights when I was confined to my house. When evening fell, everyone stayed inside. Hyenas picked through the garbage on the streets.

We catapulted from America to the spectacular Rift Valley of East Africa, accompanied by Nina Rusk, who quickly became everyone's mentor and role model. In-country training was a brilliant idea, and subsequently, the Peace Corps decided to do all Peace Corps training exclusively on site, quickly introducing would-be volunteers to the realities of working in a developing nation. After a one-day turnaround in Addis Ababa, we loaded onto a rickety bus. The next month was a lifetime of learning. We rode horses and hiked into remote areas over rough trails to conduct mobile clinics. En route north to the city of Gondar, through the high Rift Mountains, we visited one of the natural wonders of the world, the mighty Tissasat Falls, source of the Ethiopian Blue Nile and the Egyptian Nile. Later, my husband and I honeymooned in Africa, revisiting these places in my heart.

We spent a number of days at the regional hospital in Gondar, each one of us paired with a nurse mentor. One morning, an emaciated young woman, holding a skeletal infant, staggered into the hospital. The young mother had a huge caseous wound draining tuberculosis exudate from her neck. She handed me her baby, wrapped in a dirty cloth, and in Amharic softly said, "Please feed my baby. I have no milk." I took the baby, looking into vacant, suffering eyes. The baby shivered and died in my arms. The young mother grabbed her baby, sobbing and running out of the hospital. My nurse–mentor hugged me, saying, "Azoz, anchi (Be brave, my sister)."

Over many years in global health work, I have had continual exposure to tuberculosis. I have never converted to a positive tuberculosis test. However, in Ethiopia, I did get brucellosis, closely related to tuberculosis and a common problem among cattle and childbearing women in Ethiopia. When I returned to America from Peace Corps service, I received a nasty letter from the State Board of Health informing me that brucellosis is a reportable disease and that I was forbidden to ever work on a dairy farm. This letter was followed by one from the Centers for Disease Control and Prevention (CDC) in Atlanta, Georgia, pontificating that perhaps I had acquired this disease while delivering placentas in Ethiopia. They asked if I had ever delivered a placenta without gloves. What a joke! Gloves were rarely available and, if used, had to be washed, line-dried in the sun, and reused. Fortunately this was before HIV-AIDS.

One afternoon, while still at the Gondar Hospital, I decided to take a walk. I was intrigued by the rugged landscape, the small round thatch houses (tukels), and the beautiful, almond-eyed children. I wandered too far, realizing, as the sun was setting, that I was lost. A little boy greeted me, "Tenastiling, ferenji (Hello, stranger)." He said his name was Tadessa, and he asked if I was lost. I answered, "Aow (yes)." He took me by the hand and led me to his tukel. Tadessa's mother greeted me warmly, saying, "Cu-cebye (have a seat)." I sat on a tiny three-legged stool, and she handed me a plate of food, a spongy piece of flatbread *(injera)* topped with a spicy lentil stew (wat). She showed me how to scoop the *injera* into the *wat*, using the *injera* as a spoon. My mouth exploded with the rich flavor of red berbere pepper. It was love at first taste! *Injera*, made from *tef*, a small wheat-like grain rich in protein, iron, and calcium, is indigenous to Ethiopia. The grain is ground, covered with water, and fermented in a clay pot. When the yeast forms, the pancake-like batter is poured onto a flat, red-hot pan, forming a 20-inch sourdough pancake. As the *injera* cooks, the women flip it with bare hands. I tried to pay Tadessa's mother for this delicious meal, but she refused, saying God had instructed her to take care of me. Years later, days before the September 11, 2001, attack on the twin towers in New York City, I would hear this same message from a kindly Muslim woman when I was hopelessly lost in the 9,000-alley medina in Fez, Morocco, North Africa.

The month of on-site training was over. At a moving ceremony at the Peace Corps office, attended by Ethiopian government officials, our cohort was sworn into service by the Peace Corps director, an American diplomat in charge of the Peace Corps program in the country. The appointment of a Peace Corps director requires language skills, pristine diplomatic and communication skills, and keen judgment as political situations can change rapidly. When one of the PCVs negligently swam in the Nile River, after substantial warning from local villagers, he was attacked and eaten by a crocodile. The Peace Director had to retrieve the body from the crocodile (with the help of the villagers), deal with the U.S. Embassy, the volunteer's family, and the Ethiopian PCVs. He asked one of my friends, PCV Gene Hunn, to accompany him as he retrieved the body. The story of the demise of this volunteer became a widespread, cautionary tale. My children always claimed I was exaggerating the story until my daughter studied under Dr. Gene Hunn, professor of anthropology at the University of Washington. She was incredulous when Dr. Hunn told the story as an example of listening to local knowledge of the environment. He explained he was the volunteer who accompanied the Peace Corps Director to retrieve the body. Later, my brother, a professor at Notre Dame University, heard the story from one of his students, a former PCV. His student said the story was used as an object lesson in Peace Corps training as an example of active listening to local wisdom. My brother said he did not believe the story. A look of incredibility flooded his face when I told him that not only was it true but that I had been in Ethiopia when it happened.

I was assigned to teach mother–baby nursing in Addis Ababa at one of the five national hospitals. I was thrilled to discover that one of the nursing instructors at this hospital was my classmate Tenanye from Indiana University! Dejitnu, another nursing instructor with a joyful, laughing manner, would be a wonderful mentor. At a different somber and chilling time, our paths would cross again. Life took on the rhythm of work. In addition to teaching, I requested to work in the hospital with the childbearing women. As a referral hospital, many of the women were close to death by the time they were admitted to the hospital. Ruptured uteri, fulminating eclampsia, massive postpartum hemorrhage, obstructed labor, and, most of all, obstetrical fistula dominated the care. At that time, I had no idea about the ritual practice of female genital cutting, with Ethiopia practicing the most extreme and mutilating form.

The Ethiopian and British nurse–midwives were extremely competent. I longed to learn from them, and they took me under their tutorage. One day, Sister Sara, a British midwife, said to me, "Sister Barbara, you've watched long enough. Roll up your sleeves. We need some help today." As I received a tiny baby crowning at the perineum, I was appalled at the appearance of the young mother's pelvic floor, totally denuded of labia majora, minora, and clitoris. Scarified and tight, the introitus was 20% the size of an "uncut" vulva. The pelvic floor glistened and threatened to split as the baby slid into my hands. This was the first human delivery I had attended; this was also my introduction to female genital cutting. I reflected upon the ease with which my beloved Lassie had delivered her five puppies.

I became acquainted with Reg and Catherine Hamlin, two Australian ob/gyn doctors who migrated to Ethiopia to establish a midwifery school and to study ways to improve the care of obstetrical fistulas among Ethiopian women, some as young as 12 years old. In Ethiopia, the Hamlin's established the global center of excellence for the treatment of obstetrical fistula (Hamlin & Little, 2001). Their work is documented in the film *Walk to Beautiful* (www.walktobeautiful.com). Reg is buried in Ethiopia, as he wished, and Catherine, still very active in her 80s, has just been nominated for the Nobel Peace Prize. The Hamlins took an interest in me, inviting me to round with them. I carried the learning back to my students who christened me with an Ethiopian name, Tsehai, which means sunshine.

The hospitals and schools had limited resources. Even chalk was rationed! There were few books, mostly British textbooks, well beyond the English-language level of the students. There were no textbooks contextualized to the Ethiopian environment. I was learning so much and wanted to share this learning with my students. I proposed to the Peace Corps that I write a textbook on mother–baby nursing for Ethiopian nursing students in Ethiopia incorporating customs, foodways, and beliefs about childbearing in Ethiopia. The Peace Corps and the Ethiopian Ministry of Health (MOH) agreed, and with help from the Ethiopians, this effort was the beginning of my passion for writing. This project led to an invitation from the MOH to serve on the national licensure examination committee. Graduating nurses were tested for competency within their individual schools, but there was no national licensure examination. Working with the MOH national committee that developed the nursing licensure examination was a privilege.

In my third and final year in Ethiopia, the political environment in Ethiopia was becoming unstable. The power of the Emperor, Haile Selassie, was waning, and there were riots in the streets of Addis Ababa. One day, I was engulfed in a riot, the police spraying tear gas. Coughing, I hastened to the Peace Corps office which was closer than my home. Many Ethiopian university students were hiding from the police in this neutral territory. A bloody civil war, massacre, and famine, were looming. The thinly veiled account in the novel, *Cutting for Stone: A Novel* describes this civil war in Ethiopia (Verghese, 2009). The day I left Ethiopia dawned sunny in this "Land of Thirteen Months of Sunshine." My students and I had a tearful goodbye at the airport. One student, Aster, said, "Don't forget us, Sister Tsehai. We love you." I would see a few of these students again later under both happy and sad circumstances. Others would be dead within a year, providing heroic nursing care on the front lines of this bloody civil war.

My service ended shortly before the Peace Corps closed the program in Ethiopia. Emperor Haile Selassie was overthrown and murdered by the Derg, rogue forces under Mengistu Hailemariam, a ruthless dictator. He adopted Stalinist-style policies, declaring "Red Terror" (mass execution). The ensuing famine in Ethiopia was among the worst in contemporary history. Thousands of Ethiopians were imprisoned and tortured, including Melke, the husband of Dejitnu, my mentor and the joyful director of the nursing school. Dejitnu was pregnant when I left Ethiopia. A number of years later, I received a hand-carried letter, sent through friends of friends, describing her desperate situation in Ethiopia. I was able to help Dejitnu and her little daughter obtain humanitarian visas. Dejitnu, now an American citizen, passed the NCLEX and is again joyfully practicing her beloved profession of nursing. Her life has been a blessing to me, and her country, Ethiopia, is where I learned to be at home in the world.

COMING HOME

At the end of Peace Corps service, there was no preparation for reentry into American society. It was a very hard adjustment for me. Volunteers now have excellent preparation before leaving Peace Corps service as well as ongoing support with the Returned Peace Corps Volunteer (RPCV) organization. As a RPCV, I have been involved in this reentry mentoring and adjustment program. A number of my mentees have entered the professions of nursing and nurse–midwifery upon return from Peace Corps service.

I started graduate studies in public health at the University of North Carolina at Chapel Hill. The next few years were a whirl of intellectual challenge, but I felt alien from many of my American classmates. One evening some friends asked me to dinner, requesting, "Tell us all about your Peace Corps adventures." I told them the superficial part—new foods, interesting customs, the kindly people. Then the conversation went deeper. I began to describe *kwashiorkor*, the protein deficiency condition so rife among children at the weaning period, the problems with tuberculosis, malaria, and other maladies. Their eyes started to glaze over, a phenomenon I would notice again and again among my own people when they stepped into a world outside their borders. I realized that they did not want to know. Perhaps they were afraid. They abruptly changed the subject, "We've been thinking about buying a new car." From kwashiorkor to American consumerism—I was just beginning to experience "reentry crisis" as it was later labeled. Over time, I would find my people again, especially those who were passionate about social injustice and vulnerability. My new friends were international students.

I enjoyed writing my master's thesis on maternal attachment. It enabled me to visit new mothers all over rural North Carolina, interviewing them about their childbearing experiences. It prepared me for the next step in my life as a public health nurse. I nurtured the thought of studying nurse–midwifery. However, I was now married and soon would be having children. I accepted a position as a public health nurse in an innovative project, a county-funded school for pregnant adolescents as they were not allowed to continue in public school. Working in urban and rural public health was just what I needed at that point. It brought me back in touch with my own people in the geographical area where my Quaker ancestors had made their stand against slavery. I provided pregnancy monitoring and health education classes for the teens. They especially liked the classes on baby care. The teachers, public school teachers, were terrified that one of the teens would suddenly give birth at the school, although the school was located across the street from Duke University Hospital, and we had never had a precipitous birth. I offered to provide them with some guidance on "emergency childbirth," trying to help them to understand that most births progress at a reasonable pace. All the teachers showed up for these sessions!

One day as I entered the school, one of teens, Antoinette, was sitting in the hallway, shoulders drooped, her head in her hands. The young women in this school had lived their lives in poverty, and they were often suspicious of anyone in authority. The black-white color line in North Carolina was ever present. I tried to be very gentle with these young women knowing their suspicions. Very softly I asked Antoinette if I could sit down beside her. She nodded. I asked her, "What's the matter, honey?" She looked up, eyes full of pain, and said, "I just want to die."

"Do you want to hurt yourself, Antoinette?" She nodded yes. "Have you thought about how you might do it?" She nodded no. My mind raced with all the protocols and instructions about threatened suicide—72-hour hold, the psychiatric unit at Duke Hospital, and, at this fragile moment, how easy it would be to shatter all trust with her.

"I got some cookies in my office, and I'm hungry. Want to have a cookie?" I asked her. She nodded yes. Sitting there eating cookies (we finished the whole package), I began a journey with one of the most beautiful persons I have ever known. She poured out her pain, her loneliness, her hopes for her baby, her sense of despair. I did not initiate the rapid response suicide protocol. Rather, I met with her every day, and we talked. She wanted this baby; she wanted to live; she wanted to finish school. One day when she did not come to school, I was worried. Later that morning I received a call from Duke University Hospital. She had delivered a 4-pound premature baby girl the night before. Both she and the baby were doing well. I saw Antoinette one time after she went home with her tiny baby. A public health nurse followed her.

I was now 38 weeks pregnant, ready for my maternity leave. The students and I had a lot of fun being pregnant together, and I knew I would miss them. They surprised me with a shower, giving me gifts they had made in their home economics sewing class! Four years later when my daughter was in preschool, I accepted a faculty position teaching mother–baby and community health in a nursing program in North Carolina. The nursing students in this school were from poor urban neighborhoods and from hardscrabble rural areas. Over the next 3 years, I taught my assigned courses, and I designed and administered a "learning lab," a rudimentary simulation lab funded by a federal grant. One day a young woman entered my office. She had a preschooler in tow, beautifully dressed, with colorful bows in her hair. The woman announced, "I'm back." I looked at her trying to remember where I had seen her face. She pointed to the little girl and said, "This is LaTasha. Don't you remember me? I'm Antoinette." Memories flooded me as I recalled the broken teenager who had munched cookies with me.

"Antoinette, how wonderful to see you." I winked at her and said, "I've got some cookies. Do you think LaTasha would like a cookie?" She laughed and nodded as she sat down. LaTasha dived into the cookies. Antoinette did not waste any words delivering her message, "Ever since I met you, I've wanted to be a nurse. So, I'm back. Will you teach me to be a nurse?" Four years later, Antoinette graduated and passed the nursing board exam. She took a position as a staff nurse in postpartum and eventually became the nurse manager. The last time I saw her she was a busy, active professional nurse raising a beautiful child. When I returned from the Peace Corps, I had felt lost in my own country. As I worked with vulnerable mothers, babies, and students needing care and attention, I began to find my way. Antoinette was a gift to me on the road back to my own people. She was the one who brought me home.

PUBLIC HEALTH HEROES

The third goal of the Peace Corps is to bring the world to our own people. It is about sharing a vision of service and telling the stories of those who have been our best teachers, our personal mentors, and our heroes. One way this has been accomplished is with the Peace Corps World Wise School program. This is a program that provides a platform for RPCVs to talk to children's groups. When my children were small, I was frequently asked to speak in their classrooms. Often, I would receive a stack of thank-you notes after a talk. I have kept these precious notes from children just beginning to grapple with the realities of the world. One boy summed it up when he said, "I want to be a public health hero." I thought about this outpouring of his innocent heart and about the quiet public health and health professional heroes I have personally known.

One of my former graduate students, Patrice, is one of my public health heroes. Patrice is a health worker from the Democratic Republic of the Congo (DRC). His left leg drags from childhood polio. In constant pain, he uses a forearm crutch to support himself. After Patrice finished his doctoral work, he returned to his ravaged country to be a public health officer. DRC is one of the poorest, most violent, and least democratic countries in the world. Shortly after he started his position, an Ebola epidemic broke out. It takes only one infected person to spread this deadly virus as portrayed in the Hollywood film *Outbreak*. Nothing, however, on the silver screen can compare to the reality. At great risk to his personal safety, both from this lethal virus and from hysterical crowds trying to escape from the region, he ordered and enforced a quarantine of the area, saving the rest of the country and further reaches of the world from the spread of this epidemic. His is a story that we need to bring home.

Samuel is another public health hero. He was my classmate in undergraduate nursing, returning to his home in Uganda upon graduation. He was appointed to a high position as the national coordinator for tuberculosis control and eradication at the Uganda MOH. He invited me to visit his family while I was in Africa. I had a delightful visit with Samuel, his wife, and 6-week-old baby daughter. Before I left, he asked me to go for a walk with him. He obviously wanted to speak privately. When we were away from any possibility of being overheard, he explained that the political situation in Uganda was deteriorating, that the power of Milton Obote, the president, was being eroded, and there were rumors that the army, under Idi Amin, was seeking to overthrow the government. Amin had a reputation for brutality. He became a despot of Nazi proportions in the genocide that followed. Samuel confided that he feared for the safety of his family. He warned me to not contact him directly at this fragile time, while assuring me that my visit had been both welcome and supportive to him personally. When we left, he embraced me, thanking me for our friendship. I offered to help his family and him get humanitarian visas, if it came to that, and we arranged an indirect method of communication through acquaintances. That is the last time I saw Samuel. Later, I learned that Samuel, his wife, and his little daughter had been executed by Idi Amin. In the annals of contemporary genocide, the slaughter in Uganda remains one of the worst, and the story of Uganda is included in the work that my husband and I did on genocide (Anderson & Anderson, 2012).

Dr. Esther, pediatrician in Ghana, has been relentless in her campaign to protect the health and lives of girls and women in Africa through advocating for eradication of female genital cutting. When I was writing about the effect of this practice on the health of mothers and babies, she said to me, "Sister, thank you for sharing our concern for our women. Please tell everyone in the world about our efforts to stop this practice. We need your support, but we don't need governments in the West telling us how to manage this problem." How wise is Dr. Esther!

In Nigeria I worked with the United States Agency for International Development (USAID), collecting data on the implementation of the UNICEF vaccination program. Nigeria is a country rife with corruption, poverty, and unrest. It is also a country with highly capable and dedicated health professionals. The project took me to the western malarial-ridden river district of Ugbo, the northern Hausa area (a hotbed of fanatical religious efforts to undermine childhood vaccinations), and the central urban area with crushing population pressures. I worked with the health professionals on ways to overcome the formidable barriers to vaccination campaigns, including the ever-present challenge of maintaining the "cold chain" necessary to keep the vaccinations from spoiling without the benefits of consistent electricity and refrigeration. We travelled over rutted roads, frequently walking rather than riding in the bone-jarring jeep, and we subsisted on palm oil, cassava, and millet. The conditions we endured were nothing compared to the everyday lives of the people. Parents would walk miles over difficult terrain to get their beloved children vaccinated. The vaccination rate in rural areas was as high as 98% in some villages. In some U.S. urban areas, the rate is 40%.

Mabelle and Rajanikant Arole, two Indian physicians, established a sustainable community-based primary health care system in Jamkhed, located in the dust bowl of Maharashtra, central rural India (Arole & Arole, 1994). The Aroles challenged the ageless caste system, training "untouchable" women as community health workers. Their work changed the culture of this region, infamous for the high rate of female infanticide. I took my graduate public health students to Jamkhed, a 10-hour bus ride from Bombay (Mumbai) over bone-crunching roads to this outpost of India. There, we learned from the Aroles whose powerful belief in the resiliency of the rural poor changed perceptions about helplessness. While in Jamkhed, I assisted their daughter, an ob/gyn doctor, with a cesarean section. This was not a cesarean section in a brightly lit, sparkling operating room. Rather it occurred in a dirt-floor clinic as monsoon rains pounded the tin roof. A tiny, malnourished woman had been in obstructed labor for 3 days. One of the Jamkhed community health workers had convinced her husband and mother-in-law to bring her to the clinic. The baby's heart rate was audible and fairly regular, but the mother was exhausted. There was no anesthesia so the medical assistant did an intravenous valium push as the doctor opened the mother's abdomen. The medical assistant then left the surgery table to search for suture. She returned, announcing that the suture supply was "finished," but there was sterilized sewing thread. As soon as she lifted the baby out, the doctor handed me a tiny, limp baby girl. I dried, rubbed, and warmed her, trying to stimulate her breathing. A plucky child, she revived. The doctor closed the incision with thick black sewing thread. Later, I took the baby to the father and the mother-in-law, who looked in disgust when they learned the baby was a girl. I have often wondered how long that child survived in this region of high female infanticide. The Jamkhed project is a global model of community development. These most humble of people, the Aroles, left a legacy as public health heroes whose vision challenged the social order, built upon human resiliency. They changed the lives of the untouchables in this region of India.

Mayan *parteras*, traditional birth attendants, are trusted by indigenous women in Mexico and Guatemala and, even today, manage many of the births in rural areas. My husband, an anthropologist, has done years of field work in Yucatan villages of Mexico and has a longstanding relationship with people in this region. We decided to write the stories of these parteras, now a fading population as primary health care reaches the rural areas. Whereas there is a plethora of anthropological study on the Mayan parteras in Mexico and Guatemala, this research primarily focuses on belief systems and birth practices with normal birth. There is minimal work examining how these parteras manage childbirth complications. We mapped these management decisions and steps. Rich, textured stories emerged: managing hemorrhage in the midst of raging hurricanes; negotiating with inexperienced and often haughty government-service doctors; successfully bringing breech babies into the world, bringing comfort and knowledge to mothers in remote and unseen places (Anderson et al., 2004). We were humbled by their courage.

I have sometimes been asked who has inspired me. Although many persons have done so, I never have to reflect very long. It was August 5, 1998. A group of public health students and I had been in the Kenya bush for a month. The learning had been rich, and I was feeling very pleased about the success of this trip. On the last day of the trip, we were back in Nairobi, planning to leave on the evening flight to Paris. One student had a fever and another student, Alex, offered to stay with him while I settled the accounts with our hosts. Alex was preparing for an upcoming class in disaster management, reviewing the chapter on bombings. A third student, Mohammed, a physician, went into town to get some medication for the sick student as our supply was exhausted. I told Mohammed where I would be in case he needed me to help with the sick student. The rest of the students, 17 of them, gleefully took off to shop in downtown Nairobi, stocking up on elephant carvings and colorful cloth to take home as gifts.

Suddenly, there was a huge blast and glass shattered all around me as the building shook to its foundations. Black smoke filled the air. Then there was another blast. The Kenyans and I ran outside the building. Fire was erupting a few blocks away in the heart of downtown Nairobi. We heard screams. Mohammed came running up to me, "Professor, are you okay?"

"What's happening, Muhammad?" I asked. "I don't know, professor," he responded. We both started running toward the fire. I had 17 students somewhere in that smoke. I was frantic. I had to find my students. We arrived at the holocaust scene of the Al Qaida bombing of the American embassy. Simultaneous bombings were occurring in the Sudan and Tanzania. A bus had exploded, and bodies were lying charred on the ground. The American embassy had crumbled. Sirens screamed as staff from Nairobi National Hospital rushed to the scene. Where were my students? Were they alive?

Then I saw them, my beloved students, shoulder-to-shoulder with the Kenyans, ripping off their shirts to make tourniquets, giving CPR on the sidewalk, pulling the wounded away from the burning bus. It was a scene I will never forget, but what I remember vividly was realizing that the world would be safe in their hands, these public health heroes of the moment and the future.

THE CAMBODIAN JOURNEY

The story of the refugee is embedded in my family history. My journey into the Cambodian world was another refugee story, but it was much more. It was an encounter with genocide and a formative life journey that my family walked with me. There was a dearth of knowledge about this refugee population in America. Health care providers and Khmer patients struggled with profound cultural differences. Once, when I accompanied a Khmer woman to a clinic visit, the physician, in exasperation, turned to me, saying, "Speak Asian to them." I was aghast. Speak Asian? Did he not know that there are hundreds of languages in Asia?

It took time to develop relationships and immerse myself into the Khmer refugee community. I spent 5 years conducting my doctoral research at Loma Linda University, a phenomenological, ethnographic study of health care decision making among Khmer women. My study, following 30 families, examined Cambodian worldviews, beliefs, and behaviors in the management of 257 illness episodes. I conducted home interviews in America and spent time in two Khmer refugee camps in Thailand. Using participative observation, I had many experiences with the Khmer. These were busy years raising children, working, and completing doctoral studies.

In the 14th century A.D., during the period of the great Angkor kings, Buddhist monks from India introduced Theravada Buddhism, a soft, tolerant version of Buddhism. During this period, the Khmer created fine sculptures in the temples of Angkor Wat. The Mekong River, flowing out of the Himalayan Mountains, had shaped the fertile river delta. Fish, rice grown on silted river banks, and tropical fruits and spices framed a savory cuisine. The Cambodian worldview embraces harmony. Children are treasured, and the family structure easily absorbs nonrelated persons. I have frequently been told that I am an "old soul" and towoa (nonrelated kin).

One memorable event was attending a traditional Khmer wedding. Traditionally, the bride wears red and gold silk, changing a number of times into a new sarong. Each change is accompanied by the loud clang of a gong. Finally, the monk calls the bride and groom together, instructing them to sit on the floor. Then the monk calls the "angels," women who are selected to approach the couple, making "*waj*," the prayer-folded hand motions. The angels then snip a piece of hair from both bride and groom, reminding them to sacrifice and give of self to the other. To my surprise, I was selected to be an "angel" and instructed on my duties. It was the first time I had ever given a haircut, let alone at a wedding!

I did volunteer work with the Khmer refugees close to my home in southern California. One chilly November day, one of the children in my cultural immersion group asked me to explain the upcoming Thanksgiving holiday. I rattled off the Thanksgiving story—Pilgrims, Indians, turkey. I asked him if he understood. He shook his head "yes" but his eyes told me "no." During the next week, I reflected on how this story had no relevance for him in his short life of refugee camps and brutal Khmer Rouge soldiers. He and his mother had escaped the Cambodian genocide by walking through the jungle. Now he was catapulted into the world of American culture. I decided to reframe the story in an appropriate cultural context—a story of refugees coming to a new place, making new friends, and having a big potluck. We talked about the Pilgrims tasting the strange new foods and about gratitude for food and freedom. His eyes sparkled as he said, "That sounds like Khmer people. I am so happy my mother and I have food now. Can I have Thanksgiving?"

"Yes," I responded, with a catch in my throat, "You can have Thanksgiving and we are going to share this special day with you. This is now your story."

My youngest child spent many hours with Cambodian children. One year we were invited to the annual celebration of the birthday of Buddha. It was the same day as my son's birthday, and I casually mentioned this to one of the Khmer women. She became instantly alert and then got a faraway look on her face, asking. "Your son was born on the same day as the Buddha?"

"Yes," I responded, not realizing the significance.

"Will you and your son be at the celebration?" she asked. I confirmed that we were planning to be there, thinking no more about the conversation. On the evening of the celebration, we entered the home of the family hosting the celebration amidst great fanfare honoring my son as the reincarnation of the Buddha in the expression of "the white elephant prince." An albino elephant is a sacred animal, and in the Cambodian Buddhist worldview, a male child born on the Buddha's birthday is deemed a reincarnation of the sacred white elephant. My son has never forgotten this birthday party.

As I developed deep friendships with the Khmer, they opened their hearts to me, telling me about the war in Indochina and the Khmer Rouge genocide. Their stories were wrenching. The unstructured nature of home interviewing with my informants allowed me to observe the women in their own environment, but it also meant that anything could happen. Once I arrived for a scheduled interview with an informant only to discover that she was having a miscarriage, bleeding heavily. That changed the plan quickly as I examined her and arranged for her care. On another occasion, when the summer temperature was 100 degrees Fahrenheit, I entered a home where a space heater was blasting full force next to a puerperal woman. I was learning about the custom of "mother roasting" after childbirth, and I would experience this again in the refugee camps.

One informant had a sister, Sivandeth, who always sat in the garden, rocking back and forth with a distant look on her face. Each time I visited the home, Sivandeth asked me if I had seen her children. My informant told me that her sister was under psychiatric care. She had witnessed the brutal murder of her husband and two of her children by the Khmer Rouge. The other two children escaped into the jungle. Sivandeth never saw these children again.

One day during a follow-up interview with my informant, Sivandeth approached me, asking, as always, if I had seen her children and then retreated to resume her rocking behavior in the garden. The informant and I were well into the interview when the telephone rang. The informant excused herself to answer the phone, listened intently, dropped the phone, and then collapsed on the floor. I rushed to her side, asking if I could help.

"They found them," she sobbed. "The Red Cross found the children. They are in Khao-I-Dong" (The United Nations refugee camp on the Thai–Cambodian border). Sivandeth rushed into the house, hearing the commotion. The scene that unfolded between the sisters and the rest of the family was one I will never forget. I asked if I should leave, and my informant asked me to stay. I held Sivandeth in my arms, both of us crying, as my informant explained the situation to the growing number of friends and neighbors who jammed into the tiny house. As Sivandeth waited for the two children to be processed for departure from Thailand, she was a different person.

One of my informants, pregnant during my study, delivered a preterm baby girl who was admitted to a neonatal intensive care unit (NICU).

The baby was struggling, and it was unclear whether she would survive. My informant asked me to visit the NICU with her. Working in this medical center, I was able to access the NICU easily as her support person. When the informant and I entered the NICU, she whispered, "I don't think my baby will live in this life. I have named her for the next incarnation."

When I asked the baby's name, she replied, "Apsara. I want her to know that I love her and she is beautiful." In the temples at Angkor wat, the sculptures of the temple dancers are the apsaras, the essence of graceful womanhood. At the moment, there was nothing graceful about this struggling little baby whose tiny fist encircled her mother's finger. I showed my informant how to touch her baby very gently, call her by name, tell her that she was beautiful and loved. Little Aspara responded to her mother. The family moved to a new location, and I lost touch with them. I wondered what had happened to Aspara. A few years later, I was invited to the home of some Khmer friends who had some visitors in the home, including a rampaging toddler. After a joyous reunion with my friends, my host leaned over and whispered that the toddler was Aspara. She told me that Aspara had decided to live.

A significant part of my learning happened during the time I spent in the refugee camps in Thailand. Obtaining the permissions to enter the camps and do participant observation involved negotiations with the Supreme Council of the Thai Military as well as with the United Nations High Commission for Refugees (UNHCR). I was able to get permission to enter Khao-I-Dong camp, under UNHCR protection, and Site 2, the Khmer border camp on the Thai–Cambodian border. There was considerable difference in these kinds of camps. Khao-I-Dong was located about a mile from the Thai–Cambodian border and had full United Nations protection. I was authorized to interview traditional healers and midwives at the Traditional Medicine Center about Khmer traditional health practices. This data would corroborate my findings, showing that traditional practices were alive and well in California. I also met with nurses, nurse–midwives, physicians, and family nurse practitioners, who provided direct patient care and taught Khmer medical assistants in the bamboo-thatched, dirt floor primary care centers and hospitals. The camp was well organized and family units were encouraged. Many nongovernmental organizations (NGOs) from around the world provided funding and services. The government of Japan funded an outstanding project working with surviving Khmer artists and dancers in transmitting the traditional Khmer art forms to the children. Not only did this project keep these traditions alive after the genocide, but it was immensely important for the mental health of the refugees.

Site 2 border camp was the other site that I visited. It was on the border and had no international or Thai government protection. It was the first place that "displaced persons" landed in after escaping across the border from Cambodia. At Site 2, "displaced" persons were screened by UNHCR to determine if they would be given "refugee status," that is, persons caught in the crossfire, not insurgents. It was the first place where the informants in my study arrived before being moved to Khao-I-Dong Refugee Camp, then to a processing center deeper within Thailand, and finally to a "third country of resettlement."

At Site 2, I observed the Khmer practices of "coining" and "cupping," practices based upon the belief that illness is caused by "bad winds" (toxic forces within the body, a belief rooted in Ayurveda medicine). These winds had to be released either through "coining," scratching the skin with a sharp object to raise a welt, or "cupping," burning the skin by a heated suction cup. Tiger balm ointment was frequently used to ease the discomfort. It was described as painful but effective. I had observed many Khmer in California with facial scars, and now I discovered the reason for this scarring.

Later, in California, I testified as an expert witness in a child abuse case. A Khmer refugee woman had treated her sick child with coining and cupping. The elementary teacher noticed raised welts and scarring on the child and reported the family to Child Protective Services. The terrified mother, who did not speak English, was arrested and jailed. The judge released the woman, sentencing her to English language classes and child care classes.

At Site 2, I observed at a child survival center, an emergency pediatric care center, and I provided services in an adjacent home for unaccompanied minors (i.e., orphans). Many of the children were in very poor physical condition. At Site 2, I witnessed mortar shelling of the child survival center by the Khmer Rouge. Eight children were killed. Before I left this outpost of the world, I walked to the fence that separated the Cambodian border from Thailand. There I touched the fence in remembrance of all those faceless, forgotten persons who had died in the pursuit of freedom. Later, my husband and I would touch the soil at Tul Slong, the place of the skulls depicted on the front of our book on genocide, known in the west as "the killing fields."

Following my study, I obtained funding for a postdoctoral study of Khmer refugee families in Long Beach, California, in the 10th Street poverty area of the city. I continued to examine the prevalence of traditional beliefs and the impact of these beliefs on health-seeking behavior. The women described a condition called "kouchrang," which they said affected men more than the women. It was characterized by sadness, indifference, and withdrawal. The women were in constant motion, cooking, caring for the children, running the household. The men sat, many staring into space, seeing another world. Once a Cambodian man sadly said, "No one needs a rice farmer in Long Beach."

Later, after peace came to Cambodia, I was invited by the World Health Organization and the Cambodian MOH to educate the young, growing cadre of Cambodian health professionals. In the aftermath of the Khmer Rouge genocide, poverty was pervasive, and landmines continued to ravage the population. Major efforts have been made to remove these mines, one of the most dangerous jobs in the world. The great rainforests have been damaged, but there are global efforts to preserve the remaining forests. A traditional belief that supports this environmental effort is the belief in the tree spirits, the *neak ta*. While driving through the countryside, my husband and I saw signs encouraging the people to respect the trees and the neak ta. A friend, who was traveling with us, mocked this belief, and our English-speaking Cambodian guide overheard. We motioned to our friend to be quiet, but he did not take the hint. Finally, the driver stopped the car and pointed to this billboard. Then he turned around and, with a tremor in his voice, said, "You *really* need to be quiet about the neak ta or very bad things may happen to us."

My journey into the world of Khmer refugees has shaped and transformed me. These gentle teachers helped me to understand resilience. From them I have learned that peace on Earth is the greatest gift we can give to our children.

JOURNEYS OF LEARNING

Many years into adulthood, my sister and I visited the Midwestern town of our childhood. On an impulse, we stopped at the home of our first grade teacher, Mildred Salisbury. I had no idea if she was alive, if she still lived in the house two blocks from our childhood home, or if she would answer the door to a stranger. I tentatively knocked on the door. A familiar voice responded, "Hold on, I'm coming, just a bit slow these days." A stooped, gray woman, in her 80s, confidently opened the door in the manner of rural Midwesterners. I began, "I know you don't remember me..." only to be interrupted by, "Sakes alive, Barbie, how are you, child? Come on in."

My sister and I entered her knickknack laden parlor. I apologized for dropping in and she assured me that it was fine. My teacher laughed as she reminisced about my being a first grader. Tears formed in my eyes as

I thought about how the community took care of its children, grounded in the belief that it took a village to raise a child. I thought of how she guided me through the first grade reader, starting me on a journey of joy in learning.

Teachers have power to impart joy in learning. I once received a complaint from a staid professor, looking very serious, who said to me, "You make learning too much fun." I reflected upon teaching in Thailand where the students taught me the meaning of *sanuk*—joyful learning. I have taught in many sites: well-appointed university classrooms, at the bedside, sitting in shabby homes in African villages and American slums, and under mango trees in tropical heat. One exotic teaching site was in a car in an Alaskan blizzard. My students and I took refuge in this car as we could not get into the classroom building. A mother moose and her twins were blocking the entrance and the mother moose was not about to let us get close to her precious babies. Another interesting teaching venue was the lobby of a brothel in Thailand while my students and I sought cover from a torrential tropical downpour. These teaching venues happened as life happens, not as isolated events but as part of the fabric of life. They were venues that sparked joy, laughter, and sanuk.

In a field class in the Philippines, I had an eclectic group of students from various countries. We were at the UNICEF headquarters in Manila learning about child health programs. With typical Filipino hospitality, our host asked me to introduce the students but then surprised me by asking me to identify which of the students were Americans. It was a difficult moment as I noted that our host was looking directly at the White students (not all of whom were Americans) when he made this request. This was a moment of learning as life happens. I thanked him for his interest in the students and introduced the eight non-American students by nation. Our host insisted, "Which ones are the American students?" looking intently at the White students. I motioned to the remaining eight students to stand as I introduced them. A rainbow of faces bearing surnames of Nguyen, Karpinski, Ho, Johnson, WhiteCloud, Larsen, Jones, and McGill stood. I then paused and turned to our host, saying, "I would like to present the American students." Later, one of the students, smiling broadly, said to me, "That was some finesse, Dr. Anderson, and by the way, thanks, for keeping a sense of humor."

In Thailand, another group of students and I experienced an expression of Buddhist worldview about reincarnation. We had visited a temple (*wat*) where the Buddhist monks provided hospice care for AIDS patients. Their compassion for these dying patients was inspiring. At the end of our site visit, the head monk accompanied us to the door of the wat. The students were looking pretty glum. The monk addressed the students, obviously wishing to leave them with words of inspiration and hope. His words were priceless, "Your teacher is making much merit teaching you about this terrible disease of AIDS. Listen carefully to her and remember, because of her merit, in her next life, she will be reborn as a man."

My students, women and men alike, knowing my feminist leanings, could hardly contain themselves. Their faces contorted with efforts at self-control. I gave them a sinister look conveying the message, "Don't you *dare* crack a smile." To their credit, they behaved admirably until we were a block away from the wat. At that point, a number of them collapsed on the sidewalk, laughing hysterically with tears running down their faces. "Dr. Anderson, reborn a man, that will be the day," chortled one student. These students found a little piece of joy in the midst of tragedy and sorrow.

Each learner brings a personal gestalt, full of complexity and often unshared experiences. Here are two exemplar stories about unshared experiences.

Case Study 1: Unshared Experiences

Jennifer was withdrawn and distracted; nothing punctured her stoic façade until my classroom lecture on childhood sexual abuse. After class, she came to my office, unfolding her story of abuse. "I've never told anyone," she said, "but I can't keep quiet any longer." She was ready for a moment of empowerment. Years later, after accepting therapy, she has experienced joy in learning. Today she is a successful physician, married to a caring man and the mother of a little girl.

Jerry was a Hmong refugee who surpassed all the graduate students in his ability to grasp and use knowledge but whose joy in learning was waning and he was refusing help from his professors. He told me he would lose face if he asked for help. I decided to reach out to him with a metaphorical folktale from his culture which he had once told me. I asked him to tell me this story once again, as I did not want to appear the cultural expert on the story. He recounted the tale of an aggressive tiger attacking a village, targeting the villagers one by one. Although fearful to act alone, as a group the villagers decide to confront the tiger. They ascend to his mountain lair and together they defeat the tiger. I asked him if the Hmong elders ever used this story to convince people to accept the help of others. He said they did. I then asked him if the other professors and I could be his academic village and walk with him up the mountain with him as he faced this academic tiger. His sad face became transformed and he agreed to let the university "village" walk with him.

I have found that there is always a story behind each story, which enables or interferes with joy in learning.

Case Study 2: The Story Behind the Story

Nehemiah was the son of an African chief who was sent to America for education to groom him for a high position in his nation. With limited tolerance for disagreement or for collaborative work, especially when it involved female students, he experienced a lot of conflict with his peers. He was enrolled in my class, a core, required class. He advised the dean of the school that he wished to learn only under male professors. The dean gently suggested he get over that idea. He was disruptive in class and refused to turn in required course work. After I had tried multiple ways to help him, he informed me, "I don't take orders from women and in my country, we have ways of dealing with women like you." That was enough for both the dean and for me. The dean called him to his office. He was standing, assuming the body posture of the authoritarian father. Without equivocation, he led this student, so frightened of cross cultural borders, to find joy in working with all kinds of people, including his female professor!

Edward was highly critical of commercial sex workers, stating that they had chosen their lifestyle and should live with the consequences until he encountered an illiterate, hungry young prostitute with two small children on the streets of Nairobi, Kenya. This experience caused him to question the rigid worldview in which he had been raised. This transformation of reality freed him to experience joy in learning how to help others. With deep emotion he reflected on how he had been taught by this young woman, a most unlikely teacher.

Creating an environment of sanuk helps students to become engaged and transformed, as exemplified in this case study.

In many years of teaching with over 11,000 students, I have embraced joy as the transforming principle in learning. Learning happens in the context of life events and the best learning is sanuk. Thank you, Mrs. Salisbury!

SOJOURNS FROM THE FIELD

I have many stories from my public health, nursing, and midwifery work in 101 countries, including my own country. I have seen resiliency in the midst of despair, humor under dire circumstances, and the generosity and fullness of the human spirit. I will share a few of these stories.

> **Case Study 3: An Environment of Sanuk**
>
> **Tonya** was a student who had grown up with urban privilege. She stalwartly faced and transcended the difficulties of rural poverty through her ability to laugh and enjoy learning. On a long bus ride in India, she needed to void. She could not bear the idea of squatting by the road. I offered to show her how. Mustering her courage, she attempted this feat. At the very moment when I had talked her down to a point of comfort, a herd of pigs came running across a field toward the road. She shrieked, running for cover. Two hours later when we arrived at the primary health care center, she mustered her courage again, this time entering the clinic outhouse. Shortly after closing the door behind her, we heard a blood-curdling scream. Black toads were leaping out of the outhouse stall! The side of the road looked like a good alternative. To her immense credit, she not only learned to relieve herself under multiple circumstances, but she also became a strong advocate of well-placed sanitation facilities. She laughed as she described her personal growth in understanding the critical role of sanitary facilities in public health infrastructure.

Exemplars of Public Health Excellence

Finding the Lost Women: Public Health Surveillance in Tibet

As the impact of 9/11 raged across the world, I was in the Himalayan Mountains teaching the public health surveillance method of verbal autopsy to Tibetan doctors, nurses, and midwives. In the windswept plains, I taught sisterhood surveillance, a community-based epidemiological survey technique querying the local community about lost women, estimating maternal mortality where public health records are not kept and the death rate of women in childbirth was horrendous.

Messages of Hope: HIV/AIDS Education in Zambia

In Zambia, Southern Africa, health education efforts for AIDS prevention have set a standard for the world. In a Zambian village, my students and I witnessed the weekly health education drama, "Remembering the Ancestors." The air was electric with anticipation. We sat on the ground with wizened grandmothers, young mothers nursing their babies, older men, and adolescents with arms linked around each other. The drums began to beat. Suddenly the actors leaped into the center of the circle, symbolically dancing a story of love, sorrow, and responsibility. The dancers were the adolescents in the village, a part of the national youth-to-youth peer education program. A few of the dancers were missing, dead from the mysterious disease that has claimed so many lives. The dancers enacted a story of witchcraft, brilliantly pantomiming a tale about a young man who leaves the village looking for work in the vast urban slums of Lusaka, the capital. The dancers enacted the causes of urban migration: deforestation, overpopulation, drought, crop failure. They portrayed the family pleading with their young son, their only hope for family revenue, to be careful but most of all to remember the counsel of the ancestors. "Remember us, our son. Stay away from the evil women in the cities. Don't drink the strong drink that makes you crazy."

But the young man forgets. He is seduced by the pleasures of the city, and when he returns, he brings home many gifts for the family, some of them not welcomed. Soon he is coughing, getting "slim," and then his young wife and baby begin to get ill. The village adolescents were riveted to the escalating drama, reaching fevered pitch as the masked evil spirit brings witchcraft and death to the village. Then the story suddenly halts and is retold. This time the evil spirit is unmasked as the HIV virus. The drama changes to demonstrating ways to prevent HIV/AIDS through "remembering" the wisdom and counsel of traditional values. As the sun blazed overhead, we join hands and dance with joy and purpose, reinforcing the message.

Resiliency and Innovation: The Story of Bangladesh

Henry Kissinger once described Bangladesh as a "basket case." This is far from reality. Bangladesh gave the world two of the most important public health innovations of the 20th century. The first was oral rehydration therapy (ORT), a simple, home-based formula that has saved millions of children from deadly diarrhea. ORT was developed at the Diarrhea Disease Research Institute (DDRI) in Dhaka, a place of hope in the otherwise dreary, overcrowded capital, Dhaka. The other public health innovation was the Grameen Bank, the microlending approach that demonstrated that poor women could handle and pay back small loans. Muhammad Yunus, economics professor, founder of the Grameen Bank, and Nobel Peace Prize winner, created this model in rural Bangladesh (Yunus, 1999). The principles of the Grameen Bank have empowered millions of poor people globally. In Bangladesh, poor women participating in the Grameen village bank system have the best loan repayment rate in the world, close to 99%, unlike defaulting Wall Street investors.

My husband and I endured a nail-biting road trip to the poverty-stricken region of northern Bangladesh to see the "village bank" in action. We focused on recording the impact of the Grameen Bank microlending on increasing fishing resources, food security, education, and health. We witnessed a revolution of empowerment! The Grameen Bank has had a profound effect on improving the lives and status of poor women and increasing educational opportunity for the children, especially little girls. We were humbled by the resiliency of the Bangladeshi people and only wished that Henry Kissinger could have seen that side of Bangladesh.

Midwifery: The Margins of Life

Butterflies at Birth

At a small hospital in the remote highlands of Papua New Guinea, the nursing staff graciously received me, proud to show me their birthing room, kept cool in the tropical heat by open windows. Three women were in labor, quietly enduring the ebb and flow of contractions. A young primipara peacefully gave birth, attended by her Papua New Guinea nurse–midwife. As the little boy was born, a bright blue butterfly flew in the window and alighted on the shoulder of the midwife. Women are blessed in the hands of skilled midwives.

Life or Death: A Story From a Nigerian Bush Hospital

Access to timely, skilled care can be a matter of life or death. The rain pounded on the tin roof of the doctor's humble house next to a bush hospital in Nigeria. The rain lulled me into a comfortable sleep after 14 hours over brutal, rutted roads, but there would be no sleep that night. Suddenly the front door of the house swung open and Victoria, the night nurse, called urgently, "Barbara, what is your blood type?" In my sleep fog, I groused out, "O-negative," shutting my eyes again.

"Then come with me quickly," she ordered. "We need your blood." This was not the first time I had donated blood in an emergency in Africa. Many areas lack adequate blood bank facilities and even laboratory equipment to determine a safe match between recipient and donor. O-negative blood is the universal donor; it can usually be given to anyone without transfusion reaction. I ran barefooted in the torrential rain to the dirt-floor hospital.

A young woman was lying on the floor in a semicomatose state. Her husband had carried her on his back across a raging river. Dr. Elena knelt on the floor trying to stem the river of blood. Pieces of detached placenta were in a bowl next to her. "Sit on the stool," she commanded. I perched on a 3-foot stool, and Victoria inserted a needle into my arm, carefully keeping the tubing vertical to facilitate gravity flow. My blood began to pour into the attached tubing. I looked on in awe. I had heard about direct transfusion, but I had never seen one. Now I was the donor in a direct transfusion. Dr. Elena looked up briefly to say, "Tell us when you start to get dizzy." Elena, Victoria, and I worked for 2 hours that night trying to save the life of this young woman who had delivered around a separated placenta previa. When I began to get dizzy, Victoria clamped the tubing. The young mother died that night. Access to timely, skilled care, words I had frequently mouthed, now became an epiphany of understanding.

For Lack of a Bus Ticket

Many years before, I had become friends with the Mexican migrant farm workers who picked the tomato crop. When my mother and I cared for the young woman who had delivered in an abandoned barn, I knew my life work would center on mothers and babies. Now I was a nurse–midwife, practicing in an inner city clinic that served Mexican and Central American undocumented immigrants. These beautiful people had very little, but they adored their children, and they always wanted to share.

I cared for Teresa during her third pregnancy, and she returned to me, pregnant with her fourth child. Unlike my experience as a child with the migrant workers, now I could speak her language! I urged her to get dental care, as she had terrible caries. Dental caries can seed bacteria into the bloodstream and into the amniotic fluid, leading to a lethal, infected environment for the fetus. I shook heaven and earth to get free dental care for her. She tried to make multiple scheduled appointments, but either the other children were sick, her husband was able to get a day job in the line-up of undocumented workers in front of Wal-Mart, or she did not have the money for a bus ticket.

At 25 weeks pregnant, she came to see me at the clinic. She was leaking foul-smelling amniotic fluid. I arranged immediate transfer to the hospital, but little Maria Elena was born too soon and too sick. She died the next day. Her parents were heartbroken. Maria Elena died for lack of a bus ticket and a babysitter.

Cross-Species Stories

Bumped by a Goat

I had just completed an assignment in northern Ethiopia and arrived at the dirt landing strip to board my plane back to the capital, Addis Ababa. I had arrived in plenty of time as the tiny transport plane visited this remote area every 3 days. I surely did not want to miss the plane. However, something seemed wrong. The ground was littered with six airplane seats. Clutching my ticket, I started across the landing strip. An imposing man in flowing garments intercepted me. With apologetic glances to me, the local airport officials deferred to him. He announced he was the local chieftain, and he was transporting goats for his daughter's wedding feast in a nearby village. I lost that argument and spent the next 3 days fuming at this remote outpost! At least they could have invited me to the wedding!

Elephants and Buffaloes

I was evaluating a maternal–child health program in a Burmese Karen refugee village in northeast Thailand. I had ridden into the village on an accommodating elephant, until a little dog nipped at the elephant's hind legs, startling this docile creature. I plunged from the elephant basket onto the ground, looking up at the belly of the elephant as the dog licked my face. Making a quick exit from this perilous situation, I was ready to head back to the comfort of urban Thailand. The monsoons were coming to northern Thailand, and our team needed to leave the area or risk being stranded. The dirt roads would soon become a quagmire.

We left ahead of the predicted rains, but the monsoons are capricious. Within 2 hours of our 6-hour trek to a tarmac road, the rains began. Warm and lulling, I did not mind getting wet in the back of the pickup. Two other team members also rode in the bed of the truck, with the driver and one passenger in the cab. The driver looked worried, driving carefully and slowly. The shoulder was minimal and there were deep canyons on either side of the road. As he rounded one corner, the sturdy wheels of this 4-wheel-drive vehicle slid precariously across the road, heading backwards toward the canyon. In an instant, I assessed the situation and shouted, "Jump!" The team instantly followed as we leaped away from the truck bed of the careening vehicle. Later reading the book *Blink: The Power of Thinking Without Thinking* (Gladwell, 2005), I reflected on the incredible power of the mind to size up a situation and act in the blink of a second.

Decreasing the weight of three passengers probably stopped the momentum as the truck snagged on a tree with the back wheels hanging over the cliff. My teammates and I had rolled to the other side of the road, covered with red clay. The driver, wide-eyed, told us to run to the next village and get help. He and the other passenger sat absolutely still in the precariously balanced vehicle. Village men with ropes ran quickly. I surmised this was not the first time this had happened. They gingerly pulled the driver and passenger out of the truck with hand-over-hand ropes. Then they lassoed the truck bed and hitched two buffalos, landing the truck back on the road. The villagers were very kind to us, helping us to clean up and serving us a fine meal.

As Beautiful as a Cow

I love cows. They are usually gentle creatures, although I have been tossed off a few. Three times I have had the opportunity to work with the Maasai, the beautiful, unique peoples of the African savanna. Cattle herders, they revere the cow as the most useful and beautiful of all creatures. They only infrequently slaughter a bull for meat. Instead, they tap the jugular vein of the bull to collect about a liter of blood (never the cow as they do not want to weaken her), mixing it with a small amount of the cow's urine and a good amount of the cow's milk. This high protein food is kept in gourds and soured until it becomes liquid yogurt. Babies go directly from the breast to this nutrient-rich food. The Maasai craft beautiful body decorations and plait their hair with red mud to obtain the desired henna appearance. They have legends about being so fierce that even the lions fear them. The Maasai practice polygamy and polyandry, but generally within the tribe, so HIV-AIDS has been slower to reach them than other populations in Africa. Women are bartered for cows, eight cows being the top bride price and a point of pride for a woman (like a diamond engagement ring). In exchange for cows, the Maasai occasionally marry women outside the tribe.

I was visiting a Maasai village with a public health team. An elder approached our translator. He pointed to me, saying, "She is as beautiful as a cow." He announced to the men on the team that he was putting bargaining aside, going straight to the top figure, eight cows. The men looked shocked. I suggested we thank them for the kind offer and beat a hasty retreat.

Finding My Voice

I began to find my voice as a child, and over the years, I have grown in conviction about the importance of speaking to the issues of public health. Sometimes those opportunities are formal speaking engagements. Just as often, they happen spontaneously. Here are a few stories about finding my voice.

Close Encounter With a Customs Officer

It does not get much crazier than Medellín, Colombia, where I was assigned to teach a course in public health. Medellín is the center of the Cartel, the cocaine world in Colombia, and the home of drug lords. My flight and my transport to Medellin from Bogota, the capital, were carefully planned to ensure daytime travel. Nonetheless, I was relieved when I arrived at the small college where I was to teach a delegation of public health students from across the Caribbean and Latin America. The campus was guarded by dogs, and each student was expected to take a turn at nighttime armed guard duty. Medellín had the appearance of a sleepy town, except for occasional outbursts of violence. The drug lords owned the night, but peace prevailed during the day. The central market, the underground market where street children lived in dire poverty, the walled, guarded houses of the drug lords, the bombed out sites where intra-Cartel feuds were fought—the whole scene was surreal.

At the end of an exciting learning experience with these committed students, I returned to Los Angeles via Avianca, the Colombian national airline. Security was tight and inspections endless. When the plane arrived at LAX airport, U.S. Marines boarded the plane with K-9 dogs and escorted us to the immigration line. I was not concerned as my papers were in order. As I approached the customs line, suddenly there was havoc. The passenger in front of me was thrown to the floor, surrounded by four armed guards, and handcuffed. His luggage had been slashed and the white powder was found. I was next in line.

"Hello, miss," said the customs agent, "I see you have been to Burma, Jamaica, and Colombia within the past 18 months." I suddenly realized where he was going with the conversation. "What were you doing in these countries?" he asked.

I responded, "I was teaching public health to graduate students and working with a maternal health project as a university faculty."

"So tell me, miss," he continued, a smirk on his face, "What exactly *were* you teaching and how would you describe the field of public health?"

What a golden opportunity for educating the public! Never at a loss for words about the state of global maternal health or the field of public health, I launched into a full scale lecture on the state of global maternal mortality, common nutritional deficiencies in pregnancy, lack of access to safe care during birth around the world. I was really on a roll, and I noticed that other passengers in the lines were listening. The customs agent, although interested at first, now had that glazed-over look of a person receiving too much information. Limply he said, "I see you know your field, miss. Welcome home." I did not get to complete my lecture!

More Than I Asked for: Health Education in Cameroon

However, I had another opportunity to complete my lecture! I was on consultation in Cameroon, West Africa, and had been invited to give a talk. My understanding was that I was to speak for 30 minutes about the state of global health to some health professionals. As I ascended the platform and clamped on the microphone, I was informed that the presentation would be on national radio and TV and that 5,000 persons in this open air stadium were expected for the presentation. Then, as an afterthought, the Cameroon MOH host thanked me for graciously accepting the invitation to speak for 3 hours. I gasped and tried to rectify this misunderstanding, but he would hear nothing of this. He reiterated how happy they were to have me speak for 3 hours. I decided that this was a chance of a lifetime. I mentally went through the content of the public health classes I taught: Primary Health Care, Reproductive Health, Women in Development, Cross-Cultural Communication, and then, when signaled that I was live on Cameroon TV, I felt like the phoenix rising from the ashes. I never figured out how 3 hours went by so quickly!

The World Is a Small Place

My Ethiopian-American colleague, Solomon, and I were hired as consultants by an NGO to conduct a field evaluation of a maternal–child health program in southeast Asia. We planned to meet in Bangkok, Thailand. En route, Solomon began to develop some strange symptoms of ascending paralysis. He was able to contact his office, and they arranged emergency transport from the airport to an excellent tertiary care hospital in Bangkok. He was critically ill. As soon as I landed, teammates informed me of this situation. I went immediately to the hospital and was ushered into intensive care where his wife was at his side. Her back was turned to me when I entered, saying, "Solomon, are you…?" Then his wife turned to me. We looked at each other and fell into each other's arms. "Aster, why, what are you doing …?" I stammered. "Tsehai, why are you …?" she began. Aster was one of my nursing students who had accompanied me to the airport when I left Ethiopia many years before. I always remembered her parting words, "Don't forget us, Sister Tsehai. We love you." Then Solomon explained that Aster was his wife, and I was his working colleague. He asked us how we knew each other. Aster explained that this was the "Tsehai" she had told him about. Aster and I chatted away, renewing our friendship, recalling memories. She told me that I had inspired her to become a nurse–midwife. Solomon, with his customary wit, remarked, "Listen, ladies, I'm the one who is dying here, and you girls act like you haven't seen each other for years." We all began to laugh. The nurse glared at us but stopped when she noted that Solomon was also laughing, in spite of a now-arrested case of Guillain-Barre disease. I knew he was getting better! Solomon had the ability to laugh even in the face of adversity. He recovered most motor functions after rehabilitation.

REFLECTION

Much has happened since that summer day in the garden when I wrote my life goals, dreams of my childhood now woven into the tapestry of my life. Growing up in a rural, Quaker community, I made big assumptions about respect, the value of all persons, and the inherent good intentions of others. Those assumptions have been shattered by witnessing injustice, brutality, and the raw sides of poverty in America and around the globe. Yet, I have always been witness to the essential goodness in most people: cooperation, humor, generosity, hope, and desire for peace. Life has not been as simple as I had envisioned, but my passion remains the same. The epiphany for me at this stage in my journey is that I cannot be silent. I must continue to speak "truth to power" (Quaker expression), to advocate for those without voice and power.

REFERENCES

Anderson, B., Anderson, E. N., Franklin, T., & de Cen, D. (2004). Pathways of decision making among Yucatan Mayan traditional birth attendants. *Journal of Midwifery and Women's Health, 49*(4), 312–319.

Anderson, E. N., & Anderson, B. (2012). *Warning signs of genocide: An anthropological perspective.* Lanham, MD: Rowman & Littlefield Publishing Group.

Arole, M., & Arole, R. (1994). *Jamkhed: A comprehensive rural health project.* Bombay, India: Archana Art Printers.

Bacon, M. H. (1999). *The quiet rebels: The story of the Quakers in America.* Wellingford, PA: Pendle Hill Publications.

Bishop, G. (1661). *New England judged by the spirit of the Lord.* Philadelphia, PA: Thomas William Stuckey, Printer.

Breckinridge, M. (1952). *Wide neighborhoods: A story of the frontier nursing service.* Lexington, KY: The University Press of Kentucky.

Gladwell, M. (2005). *Blink: The power of thinking without thinking.* New York, NY: Little, Brown.

Hamlin, C., & Little, J. (2001). *The hospital by the river: A story of hope.* Sydney, Australia: Pan Macmillan Australia.

Henry, O. (Reprint 2001). *The gift of the magi*. Kansas City, MO: Andrew McMeel Publishing.
Stowe, H. B. (1852). *Uncle Tom's cabin*. Boston, MA: Jewett & Company.
Tyler, V. (1985). *Hoosier home remedies*. West Lafayette, IN: Purdue University Press.
Verghese, A. (2009). *Cutting for stone: A novel*. New York, NY: Vintage Books.
Yunus, M. (1999). *Banker to the poor: Micro-lending and the battle against world poverty*. Philadelphia, PA: Perseus Books Group.

CHAPTER NINE

AVIATION PIONEERS: WORLD WAR II AIR EVACUATION NURSES

Susan Y. Stevens

During World War II, newsreels narrated by reporter Helen Claire portrayed war work for women: They are flying nurses who serve in an aerial hospital service. At this Kentucky flying field, the Army shows the latest methods for transporting the wounded from the battle fields. Here's how, under war conditions, soldiers are taken to base hospitals in an ambulance of the sky. Fitted out according to up-to-date medical science....Oxygen for patients who need it...and the flying nurse is on the job as the wounded are taken for hospital care in the shortest possible time (Fox Movietone, 1943b).

This essay, part of a larger historical study to identify the images of nursing in newsreels during World War II (Stevens, 1990, 1994), describes the pioneering exploits of flying nurses. Flight nursing developed a new role for the nurse. Like the WASPs (Women's Auxiliary Service Pilots), air evacuation nurses also demonstrated that women belonged in the skies.

Two types of historical materials were studied. First, all 104 segments of Fox Studios' Movietone News footage on nursing from 1942 to 1944 were reviewed for content related to flight nurses and analyzed in the context of the times. The segments included 40 newsreels and 64 outtakes. (Outtakes are segments removed prior to public showings.) Second, archival materials were analyzed, including those provided to the news services, cameramen's dope sheets, and supportive narration cards.

The method of analysis used was historical criticism, which includes internal and external elements (Lee, 1988). External criticism answers questions of authorship, genuineness, and time and place as well as fabrications and distortions. The sources were provided by the original producer and were considered complete for the 2 years studied. Other than film being transferred to more durable videotape, the materials had been undisturbed. Cameramen's dope sheets, describing the film footage, and producer's narration cards (both available in the Movietone archives) were compared with film footage. They matched the footage transferred to videotape. Internal criticism addresses the meaning or trustworthiness of statements within historical materials. Documents are weighed in relation to truth. Issues of competence, good faith, position, and biases of the author are assessed. Credibility must be viewed in the context of the times (Lee, 1988).

The newsreel was not without faults. It suffered from a history of fabrication, censorship, reenactment, bias, and uncritical use of documents produced by the government (Fielding, 1972). Internal criticism was therefore a major focus of the study. Because choices made by cameramen and news producers had the potential to distort truth, outtakes and newsfilm shown to the public were compared with each other, with archival documents, and with primary and secondary sources, including personal accounts of World War II nurses.

THE NEWSREEL

Before television, people attended movie theaters at an average of once a week. Newsreels were considered an important component of the theater's program. Movietone News, the largest of the internationally syndicated U.S. newsfilm companies, was a major source of public information during World War II. Fox Movietone was the largest of five major U.S. newsreel companies that survived the 1930s and the Great Depression. Lowell Thomas was chief news commentator for many years (Fielding, 1972).

Movietone News had more branches throughout the world than any other news service. By 1946, it was exhibited in 47 countries in more than a dozen languages. Although the company had the capacity to produce most of its own film, reciprocal or pool agreements with other newsreel firms facilitated the sharing of footage. Government and military sources also provided film and information (Fielding, 1972). Movietone News ceased production in 1963, but Fox retained the large newsfilm library and later donated the collection to the University of South Carolina.

Criticism of the newsreels, included in later reflections concerning visual news media, revolved around the "appropriate" news to show the public, the use of recreations, the balance between news and entertainment (Fielding, 1972), and manipulation of the media by influential news makers (Rubin, 1977).

THE TIMES

General Eisenhower (1948) commented that nurses had long been accepted as a necessary part of the fighting forces. They often were found where other women were not welcome.

Chapter 9. Aviation Pioneers: World War II Air Evacuation Nurses

Before World War II, many U.S. airlines required stewardesses to be registered nurses. The nursing prerequisite was "supposed to instill confidence in passengers" (Delta Digest, 1990, p. 5). It seems ironic that men were more likely to board a plane if a woman attendant was aboard! The chief stewardess hired and trained other stewardesses, flew the first flight with new nurses, served as company nurse, checked the expense accounts of pilots, and flew 50 hours each month (Delta Digest, 1990).

In the early months after America's entry into the war, nonmilitary airlines struggled to recruit nurses against increasing competition from hospitals, the military, and industry. One advertisement, published in a nursing journal to encourage nurses to join American Airlines, Inc., highlighted the vital service to the country that graduate nurses performed:

> An American Airlines Stewardess is a technically trained and responsible member of the Flagship crew.... She is an "administrative" officer in complete charge of her section of the ship and the things she knows and the things she does are vital to efficient transportation by air.
> —Said Robert H. Hinckley, Assistant Secretary of Commerce

> Both the War and Navy Departments consider the air transport industry to be a necessary adjunct to national defense. I sincerely trust that the personnel of America's scheduled air transportation systems will feel that they are fulfilling an important duty in our national war effort and that they will continue zealously to perform this duty, subject to the call of the armed services. (American Airlines, Inc., February 1942b)

Within 2 months, the same nursing journal published a second advertisement acknowledging the "call of the armed services" and dropping the registered nurse requirement from the job description:

> American Airlines recognizes no profession more worthy of its tribute than the nursing profession, from which, since the first Flagship took the air, this company has drawn the candidates for its Stewardess Staff. American has sought among these women—and has *found*—loyalty, integrity, and competency in marked degree. Now registered nurses are urgently needed both in hospitals and in the armed forces. We have therefore discontinued the prerequisite of registered nurse training. At the same time, we have established a college education as a prerequisite.... (American Airlines, Inc., April, 1942a)

The airline's apparent patriotism in declining to further pursue nurses as stewardess candidates was also tempered by the reality that nurses were resigning in increasing numbers to pursue other war-related duty (Delta Digest, 1990).

Many former airline stewardesses would later serve as pioneers in flight nursing, evacuating wounded soldiers from combat zones. As early as 1932, an Aerial Nurse Corps of America was proposed (Kalisch & Kalisch, 1978), but there was opposition to the idea of evacuating wounded personnel by aircraft and the role of nurses in such evacuations. The resistance persisted through 1940 despite requests for information about flight nursing and tenacious efforts by nurses. Initially, enlisted men who had been taught first aid worked in bomber or cargo aircraft to transport ill and wounded soldiers. By September 1942, however, the Nursing Division in the Air Surgeon's Office was established (Kalisch & Kalisch, 1978; Link & Coleman, 1955).

A draft for nurses was not necessary. They volunteered in such large numbers that hospitals and schools of nursing sometimes had to beg nurses not to volunteer for military service so as not to deplete their personnel resources. Powerful forces in the early days of America's involvement in World War II were: increasing public support for involvement of the United States in the war; incredible changes in women's roles in the war effort (commercials highlighted "Rosie the Riveter's" contribution to the war effort); media appeals to nurses to join the war effort; and nurses' own patriotism and their desire for adventure and commitment to serve humanity (Stevens, 1990).

In return for their volunteerism, nurses gained the opportunity to practice their profession in new ways. Flight nursing dramatically improved the survival rate of the wounded. Nurses established the extraordinary record of only five deaths in flight for every 100,000 transported patients (Piemonte & Gurney, 1987).

NURSES OF THE SKY

The first U.S. air medal ever awarded to a woman was presented to an air evacuation nurse, Second Lieutenant Elsie S. Ott, for her record-breaking evacuation flight from India to the United States in January 1943 (Office of Public Relations, 1943a). She was in charge of "five desperately sick" patients and was "aided only by a ward man." The trip that would have taken 2 months on a steamship took less than a week through the air (News Release, Office of Public Relations, Bowman Field, 1943). Her personal account of the pioneering flight (Ott, 1943) described a stopover at a hospital where Sudanese ward men cared for English patients. The Atlantic Ocean leg to South America was flown by a Canadian pilot. Censors restricted information about the evacuation plane's routes; therefore, Ott's account was not shared with the public. Her travels, however, were characteristic of the lure nursing had for many women of that time. A flight nurse was able to travel to exotic climes and work with people of many nationalities. Redmond (1943), in an autobiographical account of her service in Bataan, stated that she believed nursing was the only work that would enable her to travel to faraway places. Adventure and world travel were certainly characteristic of flight nurses' work.

Ott's citation for an air medal (Office of Public Relations, 1943a) confirmed that the lieutenant's efficiency, professional skill, and unflagging devotion to duty "further demonstrated the practicality of long-range evacuation by air of seriously-ill and wounded military personnel...." The film of her award presentation by Brigadier General Fred S. Borum was never shown to the public (Fox Movietone, Army Nurses Take to the Air, March 1943a). Ott later joined the Air Evacuation Group under the First Troop Carrier Command at Bowman Field, Louisville, Kentucky.

Many U.S. Army nurses who had airline experience joined the air evacuation training program begun at that base in Kentucky. The first class graduated in February 1943 (Kalisch & Kalisch, 1978). There, nurses learned about such tropical diseases as dengue, yaws, and filaría (Office of Public Relations, Troop Carrier Command, Bowman Field, 1943b). Although not generally well known among the public, more soldiers were felled by disease than by combat wounds. A more romantic version of flight nurse training was described in a press release. A flight nurse was prepared to:

> Wing across burning African wastes to evacuate wounded from battle stations far up at the front. Or she may be flying over the wide blue waters of the Pacific, bound for some distant island outpost... (Office of Public Relations, Bowman Field, Troop Carrier Command, 1943b)

In November 1943, the length of time for flight nurse training increased from 6 to 8 weeks. Classes reflected updated knowledge in areas such as emergency medical treatment, transport of the sick at altitudes of 5,000 to 10,000 feet, the need for oxygen and methods to counteract cold at high altitudes, antibiotic and blood plasma therapies, ditching procedures, and survival training (Link & Coleman, 1955). This new knowledge added to the increasing recognition of nurses' abilities and autonomy. Flight surgeons rarely accompanied patients on airplanes. Instead, flight nurses became responsible for the care of patients until a hospital was reached (Link & Coleman, 1955).

Air evacuation was an important innovation and was given considerable attention in the Movietone newsreels. Several segments of the newsreels illustrated the training, work, and hardships involved in flying air evacuation routes. Nurses were shown receiving training at Bowman Field and at the Army School of Air Evacuation, receiving awards for gallantry, arriving on planes at airfields, and performing air evacuation work on transcontinental flights.

One newsreel showed nurses bandaging and administering plasma and oxygen while in flight (Fox Movietone, 1943b). A public relations document contained in the news film archives explained that, during flights, a nurse may have to apply splints, administer medications, stop a sudden hemorrhage, treat shock, administer oxygen, or handle any other emergency. The document claimed that "The flight nurse can do anything an MD can do except operate" (Office of Public Relations, Bowman Field, Troop Carrier Command, 1943b).

A newsreel depiction of Army nurses working with wounded personnel aboard a transport plane carried this narration by reporter Helen Claire:

> Army nurses in England are mobilized for their great tasks. Second-front invasion means many thousands of wounded soldiers to be taken care of and what a grim horror that would be without the Army nurses. They go to the battle front to do their work of mercy under fire. In France, the transportation of the wounded [is] by air and [with] a nurse on the job. Flying back to a hospital in Britain, the lifesaving plasma is administered. (Fox Movietone, 1944a)

The nurse in the scene was assisted by a male soldier. This was a dramatic change from the original stance taken by Colonel W. F. Hall, Medical Section, Army Air Force in 1939 when he was approached about having nurses participate in air evacuations. He stated that nurses were not necessary because "[e]nlisted men in the Medical Department are taught first aid" (Link & Coleman, 1955). Soon the nurses' special skills would be recognized as needed, and they would be assisted by enlisted men. Nurses increased the caliber of care aboard a plane and contributed mightily to the morale of patients who often were airborne for the first time: "The presence of the nurse quieted their fears" (Link & Coleman, 1955).

THE CUTTING ROOM FLOOR

The risks of flight nurses, said to exceed the risks to other classes of personnel (Skinner, 1981), were not given great attention in the newsreels. Nurses worked in nonpressurized cabins at altitudes of 5,000 to 10,000 feet. They often flew in C-46 "Commandos," which had two purposes: to unload troops and cargo, then load wounded soldiers at the battlefronts. The planes, therefore, were without the Red Cross insignia of noncombat aircraft and prone to interception by enemy fighters (Kalisch & Kalisch, 1978). Film provided to Fox Movietone (1944d) depicting unloading of supplies and loading wounded into C-47 "Dakotas" for evacuation in France were never shown nor were comments provided about the dangers. An account by Jopling (1990) of her World War II flight nursing experiences affirmed the dangers:

> I have heard men—even some of high rank—say if they had not seen me, a woman, on board the plane, they would not have flown on it!
>
> We carried a .38 pistol for self-protection and to help obtain food in case we were downed on an island. We also wore a cross around our neck because many natives would not harm people if they wore one. We took a knife, cigarette lighter, and Mae West life preserver most of the time also.

Second Lieutenant Mary Louise Hawkins was working on a flight loaded with casualties en route to Guadalcanal when the plane crash-landed. One patient's windpipe was severed when a propeller tore a hole in the side of the cabin. Lieutenant Hawkins kept the man's throat clear of blood for 19 hours by creating a suction tube from a syringe, a colonic tube, and the inflation tubes from a Mae West life jacket (Kalisch & Kalisch, 1978).

Comparisons between what was shown to the public and nurse's reports of their experiences show an attempt to portray nurses of the air as heroines who endured neither boredom nor too much danger. Scenes in the outtakes would have shown the public a less flattering side demonstrating danger and routine or unpleasant work. Unglamorous but necessary tasks such as spraying for protection from mosquitoes in air evacuation planes in the South Pacific (Fox Movietone, 1943d) were left on the cutting room floor. Nurses flew on planes through hazardous conditions and often on only one airplane engine (Fox Movietone, 1943c).

The enemy did not always respect the Red Cross insignia on hospitals. Bombings of medical facilities killed some nurses and wounded others. Because planes were serviced for wartime expedience, the planes sometimes seemed more dangerous than combat action. Nurses were killed or injured in plane crashes and ditchings. Thirteen women nurses and 17 men made their way by foot through the Balkan Mountains after crash-landing in enemy-held Albania in 1943. Enduring enemy dive-bombings, knee-deep snow, dysentery, jaundice, and pneumonia, the nurses cared for the sick men and each other throughout the ordeal (Link & Coleman, 1955).

The following information was provided to the newsreel company.

> The 32nd American Division ferried troops in by air, landing them in the jungle behind Japanese lines. Rations were dropped by plane, a complete portable hospital was flown in and set up in the field. All this was done through a rain of fire from Jap planes, whose attack American and Australian flyers repulsed. In addition, 100 tons of supplies a day were flown to the troops ... and casualties were evacuated daily. (Office of Public Relations, Bowman Field, Kentucky, 1943b)

A portion of Major General Hubert Harmon's speech at a military decoration for flight nurses was deleted as well as his referral to "you heroic officer nurses." The deleted portion included the following.

> There may be some glamour because you are women; some inclination to emphasize your feminine charm rather than your real achievements. (Fox Movietone, 1944c)

No public mention was made of the absence of, or later the temporary nature of, nurses' military commissions (Bullough, 1976). It was not until June 1944 that Army nurses were given temporary commissions for ranks through colonel with full pay and privileges for the duration of the war plus 6 months (Jopling, 1990). The true valor of nurses and the dangers they faced were avoided in the newsreels. Sometimes, censorship decreased the visibility of the nurses' real achievements and substituted an artificial image (sometimes presenting the feminine charm alluded to by Major General Harmon). As one historian described it, there was "an invisibility to the real nurses and an over-visibility to the image of the nurse" (Hamilton, 1993). There was also evidence that the newsreelers participated in recruitment efforts by glamorizing nursing and decreasing presentations about hardships (Stevens, 1990). It was not yet commonplace for women to be risk takers despite the examples of famed aviatrix Amelia Earhart (once a World War I volunteer nurse), or Jacqueline Cochran, originator of the World War II women pilots organization, the WASPs.

Avoided, too, were reports of the dangers of contagious and other tropical diseases to which the nurses were exposed. Depictions in the Movietone News were limited to nurses treating soldier's wounds. Descriptions of the seriousness of those wounds were sometimes limited for the sake of families, morale at home, and recruitment of other nurses into military service.

THE SKY'S THE LIMIT

During World War II, Army Flight nurses on Guadalcanal were shown being given Air Medals by Major General Hubert Harmon. Movietone newscaster Lowell Thomas described the heroic exploits and vital mission of the nurses. Harmon concluded:

> In the hearts of the Thirteenth Air Force, you are not only lovely ladies, but real comrades. Comrades who have shared our dangers and privations; comrades who have flown longer, worked harder, and complained less each day than we ourselves; comrades who have eased the pain and the suffering of many a sick and wounded soldier in this theater.... God bless you, we love you all. (Fox Movietone, 1944b)

Nurses' willingness to do more and work harder was typical of women in aviation. The need to prove themselves able to withstand the rigors of flight was something nurses had in common with WASPs and other women aviators.

Images shown in the newsreels of flight nurses were apropos of the historical moment with regard to views of women, needs of society, and stories of journalists. Nurses belonged in the skies, they were needed, and they were feminine. In a 1944 *Stars and Stripes* article, soldiers wrote:

> To all Army nurses overseas: We men were not given the choice of working in the battlefield or the home front. We cannot take any credit for being here. We are here because we have to be. You are here because you felt you were needed. So, when an injured man opens his eyes to see one of you ... concerned with his welfare, he can't but be overcome by the very thought that you are doing it because you want to ... you endure whatever hardships you must to be where you can do us the most good.... (Piemonte & Gurney, 1987)

Nurses did pioneering, important work. A whole new area of health care was developed that was to affect both military and civilian populations. Nurses' use of independent judgment in crisis situations was further developed, publicized, and accepted. Flight nurses were welcomed and were not perceived to be competing in the "man's world of aviation." Movietone News depictions of flight nurses also showed women's achievements: professionalism, intelligence, autonomy, international involvement, and technological competence.

Sharing the achievements of flight nurses was particularly important during the observation of the 50th Anniversary of World War II. During World War II, women of courage and commitment paved the way for others. Flight nurses helped the country recognize that women had a place in aviation. A new field for nurses was pioneered that demanded independent judgment, skill, and courage.

REFERENCES

American Airlines Inc. (1942a, April). Badges of accomplishment. *The Trained Nurse*, 303.
American Airlines Inc. (1942b, February). How the stewardess serves. *The Trained Nurse*, 141.
Bullough, B. (1976). The lasting impact of World War II on nursing. *American Journal of Nursing, 76,* 118–120.
Delta Digest Staff. (1990). Views of in-flight through the windows of time. *Delta Digest, 49*(4), 4–9.
Eisenhower, D. D. (1948). *Crusade in Europe.* New York, NY: Heinemann.
Fielding, R. (1972). *The American newsreel.* Norman, OK: University of Oklahoma Press.
Fox Movietone. (1943a). Army nurses take to the air (Newsreel outtake). Columbia, SC: University of South Carolina Newsfilm Library.
Fox Movietone. (1943b). In the feminine world: Nurses of the sky (Newsreel and Archival Documents). Columbia, SC: University of South Carolina Newsfilm Library.
Fox Movietone. (1943c). Medals to three flight nurses (Outtake and Archival Documents). Columbia, SC: University of South Carolina Newsfilm Library.
Fox Movietone. (1943d). United States Navy school teaches malaria control (Outtake and archival document). Columbia, SC: University of South Carolina Newsfilm Library.
Fox Movietone. (1944a). Angels of mercy: Army nurses take their place among the wounded in Europe (Newsreel). Columbia, SC: University of South Carolina Newsfilm Library.
Fox Movietone. (1944b). Heroes of the week: Army Air Force nurses (Newsreel). Columbia, SC: University of South Carolina Newsfilm Library.
Fox Movietone. (1944c). Major General Harmon decorates nurses (Newsreel outtake). Columbia, SC: University of South Carolina Newsfilm Library.
Fox Movietone. (1944d). Unloading supplies and evacuation of wounded (Newsreel outtake). Columbia, SC: University of South Carolina Newsfilm Library.
Hamilton, D. (1993). Personal communication.
Jopling, L. W. (1990). *Warrior in white.* San Antonio, TX: Watercress Press.
Kalisch, P. A., & Kalisch, B. J. (1978). *The advance of American nursing.* Boston, MA: Little, Brown.

Lee, J. L. (1988). The historical method in nursing. In B. Sarter (Ed.), *Paths to knowledge: Innovative research methods for nursing* (pp. 5–16). New York, NY: NLN.

Link, M. M., & Coleman, H. A. (1955). *Medical support of the Army Air Forces in World War II*. Washington, DC: Office of the Surgeon General, USAF.

News Release, Office of Public Relations, Bowman Field. (1943). Lt. Ott. (Archival Document). Louisville, KY: Author.

Office of Public Relations, Bowman Field. (1943a). Citation for air medal (Archival Document). Louisville, KY: Author.

Office of Public Relations, Troop Carrier Command, Bowman Field. (1943b). Air Evacuation. (Archival Document). Louisville, KY: Author.

Ott, S. (1943). Story of first long distance air transport evacuation flight (Archival Document). Louisville, KY: Office of Public Relations, Bowman Field Army Base.

Piemonte, R. V., & Gurney, C. (Eds.). (1987). *Highlights in the history of the Army Nurse Corps*. Washington, DC: U.S. Army Center of Military History.

Redmond, J. (1943). *I served on Bataan*. Philadelphia, PA: Lippincott.

Rubin, B. (1977). *International news and the American media*. Beverly Hills, CA: Sage.

Skinner, R. E. (1981). The U.S. flight nurse: An annotated historical bibliography. *Aviation, Space and Environmental Medicine, 52*(11), 707–712.

Stevens, S. Y. (1990). Sale of the century: Images of nursing in the Movietonews during World War II. *Advances in Nursing Science, 12*(4), 44–52.

Stevens, S. Y. (1992). They flew too: World War II air evacuation nurses. In B. Lynch (Ed.), *Proceedings of the Third Annual National Women in Aviation Conference* (pp. 84–91). Cahokia, IL: Parks College of Saint Louis University.

COMMENTARY: HISTORY THROUGH THE LENS OF A NURSE

Susan Y. Stevens

The Road Taken

As a nurse, I had worked in emergency rooms and psychiatry. My master's thesis was a quantitative study of maternal presence and young children's responses to emergency treatment. I wrote an article on cinema as a reflection of society's issues: "The 'Mad Housewife Syndrome': An Occupational Hazard for Women?" (Stevens, 1978). Doctoral work familiarized me with historical research and methodology. My dissertation utilized grounded theory's constant comparative analysis technique. Additionally, I had presented a paper on images of children in theater for a humanities conference. These experiences combined with personal character traits to underpin my decision to embark on historical analysis. An analytic personality, a strong liberal arts education, and a love of the arts contributed to my belief that media importantly reflects and influences society. A mother who watched three news shows daily and read the newspaper cover to cover and a father who fought in World War II enhanced my interest in World War II history and the news media.

It started with a hunch. I was teaching at the University of South Carolina when I learned that Fox had donated the Movietone News archives to the campus. Nursing was experiencing yet another shortage. There had been an enormous push to recruit nurses prior to and during World War II. I surmised that the newsreels would reflect that recruitment effort. I was curious about what help that effort could provide present times.

It was daunting to search the archives prior to computerized search availability. The librarian thought there would be little or no references to nursing in the newsreels. However, I was given permission to explore. Feeling a little like Indiana Jones exploring in the dark bowels of the library, I located files about nursing in the Movietone News archives. The files were almost 50 years old, were subject to crumbling, and needed to be handled carefully. These files included the cameraman's notes about the film made, producer's notes about what would be highlighted in the film, and historical materials gathered to underpin the film. The Office of War Information and the U.S. Public Health Service provided the newsreels much information about nursing education, nurses' work in the war effort, and the Cadet Nurse Corps. I devoted Wednesday afternoons for a year to exploring the files and taking notes. Although I was not able to take the materials out, I could photocopy some. Through numbers in the files and outstanding help from the film curator, I was able to locate and study the film segments. This also was a challenge because many of the canisters of film were stored in bunkers at the nearby Army base. The film was in danger of disintegration.

The Road Ahead

Once I gained access to all these fascinating materials, the real work began. What would I do with these archives? It was not enough to just display the newsreels. Sense had to be made of what the newsreels portrayed, what they left out, and why they were important. The newsreels needed to be explored in the context of the times, their contribution to nursing history, and also what they had to offer to today's shortage. Historical analysis was the best approach.

Was I concerned I did not have a doctorate in history? Yes. I also had been warned by a nurse historian that historical research in nursing was not always appreciated by tenure committees. Furthermore, historians did not always take kindly to nonhistorians conducting historical research. Yet, I was intrigued by the newsreels as an important and timely effort. Since World War II nurse recruitment had been wildly successful; lessons from newsreel contributions could be useful today. I also feared that time was destroying the materials.

I did possess confidence in my analytic skills and knowledge of nursing. I read widely about World War II nursing and historical research. I was able to add to this knowledge through many autobiographies of World War II nurses. *Women in Military Services* and other sources helped. I attended an outstanding week's workshop by the historian of the members of Congress. I would view history through the eyes of a nurse.

Kalisch and Kalisch (1987) used content analysis in their excellent research of media and nursing. I would also constantly compare historical evidence from primary and secondary sources with archival materials and film from the Movietone News collection.

The Movietone News worked with the government to highlight nurses' importance to both civilian and military health care. It focused on the scientific education of nurses, the humanitarian nature of the work, and the impressive innovation of flight nursing. It also glamorized nurses in a way totally at odds with the reality of the work. Although the Movietone News highlighted many nurses' achievements and challenges, the sacrifices and dangers nurses faced in wartime were minimized. The "whole truth" was purposefully concealed to ensure continuing recruitment of nurses. Although understandable in the context of the times, the disservice to nursing history was evident.

Tactics used to recruit nurses in the World War II era could be useful today (Stevens, 1994). Highlighting the rigorous and scientific education nurses receive, their technical knowhow and interesting work could enhance recruitment. Showing nurses' work at the cutting edge of health care is also an effective approach. Recognizing the importance of nurses' work and nurses' contributions to humanity are also critical components of a good recruitment effort.

I would later embark on a second study of the media's depiction of air evacuation nursing using the Movietone News archives (reprinted in this book) (Stevens, 1990). Furthermore, I worked on a museum exhibit on nursing that was displayed at the South Carolina State Museum and which later traveled to the headquarters of Sigma Theta Tau International. I also presented and published an analysis of nurses' work during epidemics, and presented an analysis of images of psychiatric nurses and the mentally ill in the media.

The Road Behind

> Two roads diverged in a wood, and I
> I took the one less traveled by
> And that has made all the difference.
> — Robert Frost, *The Road Not Taken*

What started as a hunch combined with previous experiences and personality to create new learning and challenges that I never shall regret. The thrill of exploring areas that had not been investigated before is the reward of historical study. The old adage about repeating the same mistakes when ignorant of history applies to every profession. Much can be learned from the past that can help promote a better present and future. Those who came before should be honored for their vision and courage to innovate. But first we must learn what was done, who did the work, and how those innovations came about. It is those who undertake historical research of nursing who can help the profession as equal partners with those who undertake clinical research. What helped me could help any reader who embarks on historical research.

- Build on strengths.
- Choose a subject that fits those strengths and fascinates you.
- Carve a weekly time for research.
- Continually add to your knowledge of the methodology.
- Consult experts in the field including historians, librarians, and curators.

- Read widely and, as with all qualitative methods, read more as themes emerge. For example, autobiographies of newsreel reporters helped me to understand that media.
- Interview and read autobiographies of people who experienced the times.
- Examine sources carefully. Be sure to gather all documents related to primary and secondary sources. That could include notes, memos, pictures, and diaries.
- Persist through obstacles.
- Make notes as new discoveries emerge from connecting knowledge of the times with experiences of the people in the historical events under study. Sometimes these connections happen at odd moments, even in the middle of the night!
- Know that understanding these events in the context of history takes time.
- Extend research in similar subjects and methodologies.
- Get started now!

REFERENCES

Kalisch, B. J., & Kalisch, P. (1987). *The changing image of the nurse.* Menlo Park, CA: Addison-Wesley.

Stevens, S. Y. (1978). The mad housewife syndrome: An occupational hazard for women? In H. S. Wilson & C. R. Kniesel (Eds.), *Current perspectives in psychiatric nursing: Issues and trends* (Vol. II). St. Louis, MO: C.V. Mosby Co.

Stevens, S. Y. (1990). Sale of the century: Images of nurses in the Movietone News of World War II. *Advances in Nursing Science, 12*(4), 44–52.

Stevens, S. Y. (1994). Aviation pioneers: World War II air evacuation nurses. *Image: The Journal of Nursing Scholarship, 26*(2), 95–99.

Appendix A

List of Journals That Publish Qualitative Research

Mary de Chesnay

Conducting excellent research and not publishing the results negates the study and prohibits anyone from learning from the work. Therefore, it is critical that qualitative researchers disseminate their work widely, and the best way to do so is through publication in refereed journals. The peer review process, although seemingly brutal at times, is designed to improve knowledge by enhancing the quality of literature in a discipline. Fortunately, the publishing climate has evolved to the point where qualitative research is valued by editors and readers alike, and many journals now seek out, or even specialize in publishing, qualitative research.

The following table was compiled partially from the synopsis of previous work identifying qualitative journals by the St. Louis University Qualitative Research Committee (2013), with a multidisciplinary faculty, who are proponents of qualitative research. Many of these journals would be considered multidisciplinary, though marketed to nurses. All are peer reviewed. Other journals were identified by the author of this series and by McKibbon and Gadd (2004) in their quantitative analysis of qualitative research. It is not meant to be exhaustive, and we would welcome any suggestions for inclusion.

An additional resource is the nursing literature mapping project conducted by Sherwill-Navarro and Allen (Allen, Jacobs, & Levy, 2006). The 217 journals were listed as a resource for libraries to accrue relevant journals, and many of them publish qualitative research. Readers are encouraged to view the websites for specific journals that might be interested in publishing their studies. Readers are also encouraged to look outside the traditional nursing journals, especially if their topics more closely match the journal mission of related disciplines.

NURSING JOURNALS

Journal	Website
Advances in Nursing Science	www.journals.lww.com/advancesinnursingscience/pages/default.aspx
Africa Journal of Nursing and Midwifery	www.journals.co.za/ej/ejour_ajnm.html
Annual Review of Nursing Research	www.springerpub.com/product/07396686#.UeaXbjvvv6U
British Journal of Nursing	www.britishjournalofnursing.com
Canadian Journal of Nursing Research	www.cjnr.mcgill.ca
Hispanic Health Care International	www.springerpub.com/product/15404153#.UeaX7jvvv6U
Holistic Nursing Practice	www.journals.lww.com/hnpjournal/pages/default.aspx
International Journal of Mental Health Nursing	www.onlinelibrary.wiley.com/journal/10.1111/(ISSN)1447-0349
International Journal of Nursing Practice	www.onlinelibrary.wiley.com/journal/10.1111/(ISSN)1440-172X
International Journal of Nursing Studies	www.journals.elsevier.com/international-journal-of-nursing-studies
Journal of Advanced Nursing	www.onlinelibrary.wiley.com/journal/10.1111/(ISSN)1365-2648
Journal of Clinical Nursing	www.onlinelibrary.wiley.com/journal/10.1111/(ISSN)1365-2702
Journal of Family Nursing	www.jfn.sagepub.com
Journal of Nursing Education	www.healio.com/journals/JNE
Journal of Nursing Scholarship	www.onlinelibrary.wiley.com/journal/10.1111/(ISSN)1547-5069
Nurse Researcher	www.nurseresearcher.rcnpublishing.co.uk
Nursing History Review	www.aahn.org/nhr.html
Nursing Inquiry	www.onlinelibrary.wiley.com/journal/10.1111/(ISSN)1440-1800
Nursing Research	www.ninr.nih.gov
Nursing Science Quarterly	www.nsq.sagepub.com
Online Brazilian Journal of Nursing	www.objnursing.uff.br/index.php/nursing

(continued)

Journal	Website
The Online Journal of Cultural Competence in Nursing and Healthcare	www.ojccnh.org
Public Health Nursing	www.onlinelibrary.wiley.com/journal/10.1111/(ISSN)1525-1446
Qualitative Health Research	www.qhr.sagepub.com
Qualitative Research in Nursing and Healthcare	www.wiley.com/WileyCDA/WileyTitle/productCd-1405161221.html
Research and Theory for Nursing Practice	www.springerpub.com/product/15416577#.UeabITvvv6U
Scandinavian Journal of Caring Sciences	www.onlinelibrary.wiley.com/journal/10.1111/(ISSN)1471-6712
Western Journal of Nursing Research	http://wjn.sagepub.com

REFERENCES

Allen, M., Jacobs, S. K., & Levy, J. R. (2006). Mapping the literature of nursing: 1996–2000. *Journal of the Medical Library Association, 94*(2), 206–220. Retrieved from http://nahrs.mlanet.org/home/images/activity/nahrs2012selectedlistnursing.pdf

McKibbon, K., & Gadd, C. (2004). A quantitative analysis of qualitative studies in clinical journals for the publishing year 2000. *BMC Med Inform Decision Making, 4*, 11. Retrieved from http://www.ncbi.nlm.nih.gov/pmc/articles/PMC503397

St. Louis University Qualitative Research Committee. Retrieved July 14, 2013, from http://www.slu.edu/organizations/qrc/QRjournals.html

Appendix B

Essential Elements for a Qualitative Proposal

Tommie Nelms

1. Introduction: Aim of the study
   a. Phenomenon of interest and focus of inquiry
   b. Justification for studying the phenomenon (how big an issue/problem?)
   c. Phenomenon discussed within a specific context (lived experience, culture, human response)
   d. Theoretical framework(s)
   e. Assumptions, biases, experiences, intuitions, and perceptions related to the belief that inquiry into a phenomenon is important (researcher's relationship to the topic)
   f. Qualitative methodology chosen, with rationale
   g. Significance to nursing (How will the new knowledge gained benefit patients, nursing practice, nurses, society, etc.?)
   Note: The focus of interest/inquiry and statement of purpose of the study should appear at the top of page 3 of the proposal
2. Literature review: What is known about the topic? How has it been studied in the past?
   Include background of the theoretical framework and how it has been used in the past.
3. Methodology
   a. Introduction of methodology (philosophical underpinnings of the method)
   b. Rationale for choosing the methodology
   c. Background of methodology
   d. Outcome of methodology
   e. Methods: general sources, and steps and procedures
   f. Translation of concepts and terms

4. Methods
   a. Aim
   b. Participants
   c. Setting
   d. Gaining access, and recruitment of participants
   e. General steps in conduct of study (data gathering tool(s), procedures, etc.)
   f. Human subjects' considerations
   g. Expected timetable
   h. Framework for rigor, and specific strategies to ensure rigor
   i. Plans and procedures for data analysis

Appendix C

Writing Qualitative Research Proposals

Joan L. Bottorff

PURPOSE OF A RESEARCH PROPOSAL

- Communicates research plan to others (e.g., funding agencies)
- Serves as a detailed plan of action
- Serves as a contract between investigator and funding bodies when proposal is approved

QUALITATIVE RESEARCH: BASIC ASSUMPTIONS

- Reality is complex, constructed, and, ultimately, subjective.
- Research is an interpretative process.
- Knowledge is best achieved by conducting research in the natural setting.

QUALITATIVE RESEARCH

- Qualitative research is unstructured.
- Qualitative designs are "emergent" rather than fixed.
- The results of qualitative research are unpredictable (Morse, 1994).

KINDS OF QUALITATIVE RESEARCH

- Grounded theory
- Ethnography (critical ethnography, institutional ethnography, ethnomethodology, ethnoscience, etc.)
- Phenomenology
- Narrative inquiry
- Others

CHALLENGES FOR QUALITATIVE RESEARCHERS

- Developing a solid, convincing argument that the study contributes to theory, research, practice, and/or policy (the "so what?" question)
- Planning a study that is systematic, manageable, and flexible (to reassure skeptics):
  - Justification of the selected qualitative method
  - Explicit details about design and methods, without limiting the project's evolution
  - Attention to criteria for the overall soundness or rigor of the project

QUESTIONS A PROPOSAL MUST ANSWER

- Why should anyone be interested in my research?
- Is the research design credible, achievable, and carefully explained?
- Is the researcher capable of conducting the research? (Marshall & Rossman, 1999)

TIPS TO ANSWER THESE QUESTIONS

- Be practical (practical problems cannot be easily brushed off)
- Be persuasive ("sell" your proposal)
- Make broad links (hint at the wider context)
- Aim for crystal clarity (avoid jargon, assume nothing, explain everything) (Silverman, 2000)

SECTIONS OF A TYPICAL QUALITATIVE PROPOSAL

- Introduction
  - Introduction of topic and its significance
  - Statement of purpose, research questions/objectives
- Review of literature
  - Related literature and theoretical traditions
- Design and methods
  - Overall approach and rationale
  - Sampling, data gathering methods, data analysis
  - Trustworthiness (soundness of the research)
  - Ethical considerations
- Dissemination and knowledge translation
  - Timeline
  - Budget
  - Appendices

INTRODUCING THE STUDY—FIRST PARA

- Goal: Capture interest in the study
  - Focus on the importance of the study (Why bother with the question?)
  - Be clear and concise (details will follow)
  - Provide a synopsis of the primary target of the study
  - Present persuasive logic backed up with factual evidence

THE PROBLEM/RESEARCH QUESTION

- The problem can be broad, but it must be specific enough to convince others that it is worth focusing on.
- Research questions must be clearly delineated.
- The research questions must sometimes be delineated with sub-questions.
- The scope of the research question(s) needs to be manageable within the time frame and context of the study.

PURPOSE OF THE QUALITATIVE STUDY

- Discovery?
- Description?
- Conceptualization (theory building)?
- Sensitization?
- Emancipation?
- Other?

LITERATURE REVIEW

- The literature review should be selective and persuasive, building a case for what is known or believed, what is missing, and how the study fits in.
- The literature is used to demonstrate openness to the complexity of the phenomenon, rather than funneling toward an a priori conceptualization.

METHODS—CHALLENGES HERE

- Quantitative designs are often more familiar to reviewers.
- Qualitative researchers have a different language.

METHODS SECTION

- Orientation to the method:
  - Description of the particular method that will be used and its creators/interpreters
  - Rationale for qualitative research generally and for the specific method to be used

QUALITATIVE STUDIES ARE VALUABLE FOR RESEARCH

- It delves deeply into complexities and processes.
- It focuses on little-known phenomena or innovative systems.

- It explores informal and unstructured processes in organizations.
- It seeks to explore where and why policy and local knowledge and practice are at odds.
- It is based on real, as opposed to stated, organizational goals.
- It cannot be done experimentally for practical or ethical reasons.
- It requires identification of relevant variables (Marshall & Rossman, 1999).

SAMPLE

- Purposive or theoretical sampling
  - The purpose of the sampling
  - Characteristics of potential types of persons, events, or processes to be sampled
  - Methods of making decisions about sampling
- Sample size
  - Estimates provided based on previous experience, pilot work, etc.
- Access and recruitment

DATA COLLECTION AND ANALYSIS

- Types: Individual interviews, participant observation, focus groups, personal and public documents, Internet-based data, videos, and so on, all of which vary with different traditions.
- Analysis methods vary depending on the qualitative approach.
- Add DETAILS and MORE DETAILS about how data will be gathered and processed (procedures should be made public).

QUESTIONS FOR DATA MANAGEMENT AND ANALYSIS

- How will data be kept organized and retrievable?
- How will data be "broken up" to see something new?
- How will the researchers engage in reflexivity (e.g., be self-analytical)?
- How will the reader be convinced that the researcher is sufficiently knowledgeable about qualitative analysis and has the necessary skills?

TRUSTWORTHINESS (SOUNDNESS OF THE RESEARCH)

- Should be reflected throughout the proposal
- Should be addressed specifically, with the relevant criteria for the qualitative approach used
- Should provide examples of the strategies used:
  - Triangulation
  - Prolonged contact with informants, including continuous validation of data
  - Continuous checking for representativeness of data and fit between coding categories and data
  - Use of expert consultants

EXAMPLES OF STRATEGIES FOR LIMITING BIAS IN INTERPRETATIONS

- Planning to search for negative cases
- Describing how analysis will include a purposeful examination of alternative explanations
- Using members of the research team to critically question the analysis
- Planning to conduct an audit of data collection and analytic strategies

OTHER COMPONENTS

- Ethical considerations
  - Consent forms
  - Dealing with sensitive issues
- Dissemination and knowledge translation
- Timeline
- Budget justification

LAST BITS OF ADVICE

- Seek assistance and pre-review from others with experience in grant writing (plan time for rewriting).
- Highlight match between your proposal and purpose of competition.
- Follow the rules of the competition.
- Write for a multidisciplinary audience.

REFERENCES

Marshall, C., & Rossman, G. B. (1999). *Designing qualitative research*. Thousand Oaks, CA: Sage.

Morse, J. M. (1994). Designing funded qualitative research. In N. Denzin & Y. Lincoln (Eds.), *Handbook of qualitative research* (pp. 220–235). Thousand Oaks, CA: Sage.

Silverman, D. (2000). *Doing qualitative research*. Thousand Oaks, CA: Sage.

Appendix D

Outline for a Research Proposal

Mary de Chesnay

The following guidelines are meant as a general set of suggestions that supplement the instructions for the student's program. In all cases where there is conflicting advice, the student should be guided by the dissertation chair's instructions. The outlined plan includes five chapters: the first three constitute the proposal and the remaining two the results and conclusions, but the number may vary depending on the nature of the topic or the style of the committee chair (e.g., I do not favor repeating the research questions at the beginning of every chapter, but some faculty do. I like to use this outline but some faculty prefer a different order. Some studies lend themselves to four instead of five chapters.).

Chapter I: Overview of the Study (or Preview of Coming Attractions) is a few pages that tell the reader:

- What he or she is going to investigate (purpose or statement of the problem and research questions or hypotheses).
- What theoretical support the idea has (conceptual framework or theoretical support). In qualitative research, this section may include only a rationale for conducting the study, with the conceptual framework or typology emerging from the data.
- What assumptions underlie the problem.
- What definitions of terms are important to state (typically, these definitions in quantitative research are called *operational definitions* because they describe how one will know the item when one sees it. An operational definition usually starts with the phrase: "a score of ... or above on the [name of instrument]"). One may also want to include a conceptual definition, which is the usual meaning of the concept of interest or a definition according to a specific author. In contrast, qualitative research usually does not include measurements, so operational definitions are not appropriate, but conceptual definitions may be important to state.

- What limitations to the design are expected (not delimitations, which are intentional decisions about how to narrow the scope of one's population or focus).
- What the importance of the study (significance) is to the discipline.

Chapter II: The Review of Research Literature (or Why You Are Not Reinventing the Wheel)

For Quantitative Research:
Organize this chapter according to the concepts in the conceptual framework in Chapter I and describe the literature review thoroughly first, followed by the state of the art of the literature and how the study fills the gaps in the existing literature. Do not include non research literature in this section—place it in Chapter I as introductory material if the citation is necessary to the description.

- Concept 1: a brief description of each study reviewed that supports concept 1 with appropriate transitional statements between paragraphs
- Concept 2: a brief description of each study reviewed that supports concept 2 with appropriate transitional statements between paragraphs
- Concept 3: a brief description of each study reviewed that supports concept 3 with appropriate transitional statements between paragraphs
- And so on, for as many concepts as there are in the conceptual framework (I advise limiting the number of concepts for a master's degree thesis owing to time and cost constraints)
- Areas of agreement in the literature—a paragraph, or two, that summarizes the main points on which authors agree
- Areas of disagreement—where the main issues on which authors disagree are summarized
- State of the art on the topic—a few paragraphs in which the areas where the literature is strong and where the gaps are, are clearly articulated
- A brief statement of how the study fills the gaps or why the study needs to be conducted to replicate what someone else has done

For Qualitative Research:
The literature review is usually conducted after the results are analyzed and the emergent concepts are known. The literature may then be placed in Chapter II of the proposal as shown earlier or incorporated into the results and discussion.

Chapter III: Methodology (or Exactly What You Are Going to Do Anyway)

- Design (name the design—e.g., ethnographic, experimental, survey, cross-sectional, phenomenological, grounded theory, etc.).
- Sample—describe the number of people who will serve as the sample and the sampling method: Where and how will the sample be recruited? Provide the rationale for sample selection and methods. Include the institutional review board (IRB) statement and say how the rights of subjects (Ss) will be protected, including how informed consent will be obtained and the data coded and stored.
- Setting—where will data collection take place? In quantitative research, this might be a laboratory or, if a questionnaire, a home. If qualitative, there are special considerations of privacy and comfortable surroundings for the interviews.
- Instruments and data analysis—how will the variables of interest be measured and how will sense be made of the data, if quantitative, and if qualitative, how will the data be coded and interpreted—that is, for both, this involves how the data will be analyzed.
- Validity and reliability—how will it be known if the data are good (in qualitative research, these terms are "accuracy" and "replicability").
- Procedures for data collection and analysis: a 1-2-3 step-by-step plan for what will be done.
- Timeline—a chart that lists the plan month by month—use Month 1, 2, 3 instead of January, February, March.

The above three-chapter plan constitutes an acceptable proposal for a research project. The following is an outline for the final two chapters.

Chapter IV: Results (What I Discovered)

- Some researchers like to describe the sample in this section as a way to lead off talking about the findings.
- In the order of each hypothesis or research question, describe the data that addressed that question. Use raw data only; do not conclude anything about the data and make no interpretations.

Chapter V: Discussion (or How I Can Make Sense of All This)

- Conclusions—a concise statement of the answer to each research question or hypothesis. Some people like to interpret here—that is, to say how confident they can be about each conclusion.

- Implications—how each conclusion can be used to help address the needs of vulnerable populations or nursing practice, education, or administration.
- Recommendations for further research—that is, what will be done for an encore?

Index

Abel, Emily K., 31
Abel-Smith, Brian, 29
Adelphi Archives, 50
Allende, Salvador, 80–81
American Association for the History of Nursing (AAHN), 3
American Nursing: A History of Knowledge, Authority and the Meaning of Work, 6
American Nursing History Archives, 34
American Red Cross, 5
Armeny, Susan, 28
Arole, Mabelle, 154
Arole, Rajanikant, 154
Ashley, Ashley, 25–26
Austin, Annie L., 33

Baly, Monica, 26
Barbara Bates Center for the Study of Nursing, 12
Beck, Cheryl Tatono, 6
Bellevue Alumnae Center for Nursing in Guilderland, 12
Birnbach, Nettie, 3, 15, 18, 54
Bolton Act, 51
Borum, Brigadier General Fred S., 179
Boschma, Gertje, 48
Bostridge, Mark, 27
Brodie, Barbara, 3, 32, 52
Bronx Community College (BCC), 42–43
Brown, Janie, 15
Brown, Thomas, 31

Brush, Barbara, 29, 31
Buck, Joy, 48
Buhler-Wilkerson, Karen, 31, 33
Bullough, Bonnie, 3, 26
Bullough, Vern, 3, 26, 32

Calabria, Michael, 27
Canadian Association for the History of Nursing (CAHN), 3
Carnegie, M. Elizabeth, 29
Carnochan, Doug, 98–100
"Celluloid Angels" study. *See also* nurses
  challenges and issues, 115–117
  nursing and nurses portrayed in, 107–108, 111–114
  qualitative analysis of themes, 109–111
Chesler, Ellen, 31
Chilean nursing, 77–79
Choy, Catherine Cenzia, 29
Christy, Theresa, 3, 33, 47
City University of New York (CUNY), 42
Claire, Helen, 180
Columbia University Gottesman Library, 49
community mental health care
  experiences, 86
  study. *See also* public health nursing
    conceptualizing the study, 87–91
    oral history research, 91–96
    summary, 87
Connolly, Cynthia, 6, 17, 31, 51

D'Antonio, Patricia, 4–6, 50–51
Davis, Thadious, 31
Dineh (Navajo people), health care of
    background, 122–124
    cross-cultural strengths, 127–130
    cultural contexts of health and illness, 132–133
    Forster's therapeutic presence *vs* Navajo healing system, 127–130
    hazardous effects on Navajo culture, 130–132
    Navajo healers, role of, 129, 132
    Navajo Reservation, context of health services, 124–127
Dock, Lavinia L., 20
Dolan, Josephine, 25

Eisenhower, D.D. (General), 176
Eleanor Crowder Bjoring Center for Nursing Historical Inquiry at the University of Virginia in Charlottesville, 12
essays
    American Nurses in Fiction: An Anthology of Short Stories, 33
    American Nursing: A Biographical Dictionary, 32
    American Nursing: From Hospitals to Health Care Systems, 31
    American Nursing History Archives, 34
    And If I Perish: Frontline U.S. Army Nurses in World War II, 30
    An Officer and a Lady: Canadian Military Nursing and the Second World War, 30
    articles published in journals, 23
    Bedside Matters: The Transformation of Canadian Nursing, 29
    Black Women in White: Racial Conflict and Cooperation in the Nursing Profession, 1890–1950, 28
    Bodies and Souls: Politics and the Professionalization of Nursing in France, 1880–1922, 29
    Cassandra, 27
    Clara Barton: Professional Angel, 31
    Cornerstone for Nursing Education, a History of the Division of Nursing Education of Teachers College, Columbia University, 1899–1947, 33
    Devices and Desires: Gender, Technology, and American Nursing, 30
    Dictionary of American Nursing Biography, 32
    Divided Sisterhood: Race, Class and Gender in the South African Nursing Profession, 29
    Dorothea Dix: New England Reformer, 31
    The East Harlem Health Center Demonstration: An Anthology of Pamphlets, 33
    Empire of Care: Nursing and Migration in Filipino American History, 29
    Ever Yours, Florence Nightingale: Selected Letters, 27
    False Dawn: The Rise and Decline of Public Health Nursing, 1900–1930, 31
    Feminism and Nursing: An Historical Perspective on Power, Status, and Political Activism in the Nursing Profession, 26
    Florence Nightingale: Avenging Angel, 26
    Florence Nightingale: Letters From the Crimea, 27
    Florence Nightingale: Reputation and Power, 26
    Florence Nightingale: The Making of an Icon, 27
    Florence Nightingale and Her Era: A Collection of New Scholarship, 26
    Florence Nightingale and the Health of the Raj, 26
    Florence Nightingale and the Nursing Legacy, 26
    Healer from the Outback: Sister Elizabeth Kenny, Polio and American Medicine, 1940–1952, 31
    Hearts of Wisdom: American Women Caring for Kin, 1850–1940, 31

A History of Apprenticeship Nurse Training in Ireland: Bright Faces and Neat Dresses, 29
A History of Nursing, 23–25
A History of Nursing Sourcebook, 33
In Search of Nella Larsen: A Biography of the Color Line, 31
Lamps of the Prairie: A History of Nursing in Kansas, 32
Lillian Wald: A Biography, 32
Lucy Osburn, A Lady Displaced: Florence Nightingale's Envoy to Australia, 32
Making Room in the Clinic: Nurse Practitioners and the Evolution of Modern Health Care, 30
Mary Breckinridge: The Frontier Nursing Service & Rural Health in Appalachia, 32
Mary Seacole: The Most Famous Black Woman of the Victorian Age, 31
Medical Women and Victorian Fiction, 26
A Midwife's Tale: The Life of Martha Ballard, Based on Her Diary, 1785–1812, 31
Mr. Jefferson's Nurses: The University of Virginia School of Nursing, 1901–2001, 32
Nella Larsen, Novelist of the Harlem Renaissance: A Woman's Life Unveiled, 31
Nightingales: The Extraordinary Upbringing and Curious Life of Miss Florence Nightingale, 26
No Place Like Home: A History of Nursing and Home Care in the United States, 31
Notes on Nursing, Notes on Hospitals, 27
No Time for Prejudice; A Story of the Integration of Negroes in Nursing in the United States, 29
Nurses in Nazi Germany: Moral Choice in History, 29–30
Nurses of All Nations: A History of the International Council of Nurses, 1899–1999, 29
Nursing and the Privilege of Prescription, 1893–2000, 30
Nursing and the Public's Health: An Anthology of Sources, 33
Nursing, Physician Control, and the Medical Monopoly, 26
Ordered to Care: The Dilemma of American Nursing, 1850–1945, 28
The Origins and Rise of Associate Degree Nursing Education, 33
Pathfinders: A History of the Progress of Colored Graduate Nurses, 28
The Path We Tread: Blacks in Nursing Worldwide, 1854–1994, 29
"The Physician's Hand": Work Culture and Conflict in American Nursing, 28
primary, 11–13
on professionalism, 28
Promise on Parnassus: The First Century of the UCSF School of Nursing, 32
Saving Sickly Children: The Tuberculosis Preventorium in American Life, 1909–1970, 31
Say Little, Do Much: Nurses, Nuns, and Hospitals in the Nineteenth Century, 31
secondary, 10–11
Suggestions for Thought by Florence Nightingale: Selections and Commentaries, 27
theme of subordination, 25
Uneven Developments: The Ideological Work of Gender in Mid-Victorian England, 25–26
Unlikely Entrepreneurs: Catholic Sisters and the Hospital Marketplace, 1865–1925, 31
We Band of Angels: The Untold Story of American Nurses Trapped on Bataan by the Japanese, 30
Woman of Valor: Margaret Sanger and the Birth Control Movement in America, 31
Women at the Front: Hospital Workers in Civil War America, 30

"ethical acceptability" of a proposed research project, 15–16
European Nursing History Group (ENHG), 3

Fairman, Julie, 4–6, 10, 30, 51
Farrell, Ray, 98–100
Fealy, Gerard, 29
Feld, Marjorie, 32
field stories, public health nursing, 165
   encounter with a customs officer, 171
   finding my voice, 170–172
   health education in Cameroon, 172
   HIV/AIDS education in Zambia, 165–166
   Maasai community, working with, 170
   maternal–child health program, Thailand, 169–170
   maternal–child health program in southeast Asia, 172–173
   midwifery, Papua New Guinea, 167
   midwifery care for Mexican and Central American immigrants, 168
   oral rehydration therapy, Bangladesh, 166
   skilled care, Nigeria, 167–168
   surveillance in Tibet, 165
films and movies, 106–107. *See also* nurses; oral histories
   depiction of Army nurses, 180, 183
   newsreels, 176
   nursing and nurses portrayed in, 107–108, 111–114
   personal reflection, 117
   qualitative analysis of themes, 109–111
Fitzpatrick, Louise, 3, 47
Flood, Marilyn, 32
"Focker" films, 107
Fondiller, S., 18
Forster, Elizabeth, 133
Frontier Nursing Service, 5

Gibson, Mary, 52
Gill, Gillian, 26
Gilpin, Laura, 122, 133
Goan, Melanie Beals, 32
Godden, Judith, 32
Goldie, Sue, 27
Gourlay, Jharna, 26
Grympa, Sonya, 48

Haase, Patricia, 33
Hall, W. F. (Colonel), 180
Hamilton, Diane, 21
Hampton, Isabel, 28
Harmon, Hubert (Major General), 182–183
Hawkins, Mary Louise, 181
Henderson, Virginia, 44
Henry Street Nurses' Settlement House, 5
Hiestand, Wanda, 15
Hine, Darlene Clark, 28–29, 33
historical criticism, 175–176
historical research
   advantages of learning, 1
   becoming a historian, 4
   case studies, use of, 4–5
   covering the cost of, 17
   ethical concerns, 15
   institutional review board (IRB) approval, 15–16
   modern technology and, 34
   published work on, 6
   during 1960s and 1970s, 2–3
   steps of. *see* steps in historical research
   time constraints, 17–19
   value of, 2–6
The Histories (Herodotus), 105–106
A History of Nursing, 21
Hutchinson, George, 31

institutional review board (IRB) approval, 15–16
James, Janet Wilson, 28

Kalish, Beatrice J., 25
Kalish, Philip A., 25
Kaufman, Martin, 32
Keeling, Arlene, 4, 6, 30, 48, 52

Larsen, Nella, 31
Lewenson, Sandy, 4–5, 47
Lynaugh, Joan, 3–4, 8, 14, 29–31, 51
Lyons, Larry, 97

Macrae, Janet, 27
Madison, Ellen, 98
Maggs, Christopher, 4, 29
Making Room in the Clinic: Nurse Practitioners and the Evolution of Modern Health Care, 6
malnutrition problem, in Chile, 74
Marks, Shula, 29
McAllister, Annemarie, 1
McDonald, Lynn, 27
McFarland-Icke, Bronwyn Rebekah, 30
McManus, R. Louise, 8, 41, 44–47, 55–56
McPherson, Katherine, 29
Melli, Sheila, 44
Melosh, Barbara, 28
Monahan, Evelyn, 30
Montag, Mildred, 8, 42, 44–47, 51, 55–56
Moore, Judith, 29

Neidel-Greenlee, Rosemary, 30
Nelson, Sioban, 31
Nergaard, Bea, 27
Newton, M.E., 19
Nightingale, Florence, 24–28, 32
Notter, Lucille, 2–3
nurse historian, becoming a
  collegial networking, 46–47
  communication with committee members, 54
  cost of doing research, 52–53
  developing an interest in history, 43–44
  exploration of archives, 49–52
  exposure to other nurse historians, 47
  learning historical method, 48–55
  lessons learned, 55–56
  networking with historians, 48
  stopping the research, 54–55
  timeframe and contexts, 53–54
  value of historical research, 44–46
nurse practitioner movement, 10
nurses
  air evacuation nurse, 178–180
  in armed forces, 176–178
  Army Flight, 183–184
  historians, 1. *see also* nurse historian, becoming a
  perception of history, 186–189
  risks of flight nurses, 180–182
  as stewardess candidates, 177–178
Nurses on the Front Line: When Disaster Strikes 1870–2010, 6
Nurse Training Act of 1943, 51
nursing and nurses, portrayed in films,
  challenges to study, 115–117
  qualitative analysis of themes, 109–111
  study design, 107–108
  study results, 109–111
  as heroines in romantic roles or as self-sacrificial careers, 111, 113–114
  as sex objects, 111–113
Nursing and the Privilege of Prescription, 1893–2000, 6
nursing education, 1
nursing history dissertation, organization of
  archive considerations, 70
  choosing a committee, 65–68
  choosing a topic of interest, 61–62
  corroborating evidence, 73
  footnotes or endnotes, 73–76
  grants and funding, 68–70
  introduction, 60
  organizing resources, 62–64
  Rockefeller Foundation's nurse leader, 70–72
  setting the time period, 76–79
  translation of documents, 79–83
Nursing History Review, 23
Nursing Inquiry, 23
Nursing Interventions Through Time: History as Evidence, 6

nursing journals, 191–193
Nutting, M. Adelaide, 20, 23–24, 42

oral histories, 13, 91–96. *See also* films and movies
  analysis and interpretation of, 96–100
  collecting oral histories and consent, 95–96
  memories, 91–94
  preservation, 96
  recruitment and sampling of interviewees, 94–95
Ott, Elsie S., 178–179

Paden, Rose, 74
Peplau, Hildegard, 44
Poovey, Mary, 25
prenatal care, 74
primary sources, for historical research, 11–13
Pryor, Elizabeth, 31
public health nursing. *See also* community mental health care, study
  cross-cultural context of, 121–122. *See also Dineh* (Navajo people), health care of
  early 20th century, 122
  mentors and heroes, 152–156

qualitative data analysis, 105–106
qualitative proposal
  elements of, 195–196
  writing a, 197–202
quantitative research, 3

Rafferty, Anne Marie, 29
refugees, stories of
  battling of epidemics, 140
  infant mortality, 140–141
  Irish American refugees, 137–142
  Khmer refugee community, 156–161
  Ku Klux Klan, persecution by, 141–142
  Midwestern life, 142–144, 161–163
  Peace Corps service, 144–149

Quakers, 138–139
Returned Peace Corps Volunteer (RPCV) organization, 149–152
Society of Friends, 138
unshared experiences, 163
research proposal, outline for, 205–208
Reverby, Susan, 28, 33
Riglosa, Elaine LaMonica, 47
RN-BSN program, 46
Roberts, Joan, 26
Roberts, Mary, 25
Robinson, Jane, 31
Robinson, Victor, 25
Rockefeller, Mary, 45
Rockefeller Archives, 49–50, 62
Rogers, Martha, 44
Rogers, Naomi, 31
Routledge Handbook of the Global History of Nursing, 4
Routledge International Handbook of Qualitative Nursing Research, 6
rural public health nursing service, 5

Sandelowski, Margarete, 30
Saving Sickly Children: The Tuberculosis Preventorium in American Life, 1909–1970, 6
Schultheiss, Katrin, 29
Schultz, Jane, 30
secondary sources for historical research, 10–11
Shopes, L. (n.d.), 16
Shyrock, Richard, 25
Small, Hugh, 26
Smith, F. B., 26
Speakman, Elizabeth, 47
Stanton, Marietta, 26
Staupers, Mabel, 28
steps in historical research
  area of interest, 7–8
  consent for participation, 16
  data interpretation, 13–14
  dissemination of results, 19
  ethics, 14–16
  literature search, 10

oral histories, 13
primary source materials, 11–13
questions, choosing, 8–9
secondary source materials, 10–11
selection of doctoral committee advisor or a mentor, 18
telling the story, 14
title determination, 9–10
Stewart, Isabel Maitland, 42
Swenson, Kristine, 26

Tagliareni, Elaine, 47
Tennant, Mary Elizabeth, 70–71
Thetis Group, 26
Thomas, Lowell, 176, 183
Thoms, Adah, 28

Toman, Cynthia, 30

Vicinus, Martha, 27
Wald, Lillian, 5
Wall, Barbra Mann, 6, 31, 51
    advice to nurses, 40
    on current trends in historical research, 39
    sources for historical research, 40
Whelan, Jean, 4, 17, 51
Woodham-Smith, Cecil, 26
World War II, role of nurses, 176–178
Writers' Program (part of WPA), 32–33

Zotero, 17, 64

Made in the USA
Monee, IL
13 September 2025